Forensic aspects in emergency medicine

Sieglinde Ahne • Thomas Ahne
Michael Bohnert

Forensic aspects in emergency medicine

For Ambulance- and Emergency Physician

Springer

Sieglinde Ahne
Institut für Rechtsmedizin
University Medical Center
Freiburg
Freiburg im Breisgau, Baden-Württemberg, Germany

Thomas Ahne
Gesundheitszentrum Todtnau
Todtnau, Baden-Württemberg,
Germany

Michael Bohnert
Institut f. Rechtsmedizin
University of Würzburg
Würzburg, Germany

ISBN 978-3-662-65948-9 ISBN 978-3-662-65949-6 (eBook)
https://doi.org/10.1007/978-3-662-65949-6

Cover illustration: (c) SZ-Designs/stock.adobe.com//cover design: deblik Berlin

This Springer imprint is published by the registered company Springer-Verlag GmbH, DE, part of Springer Nature.
The registered company address is: Heidelberger Platz 3, 14197 Berlin, Germany

Preface to the Second Edition

Ten years later, much has changed and much has remained. We have remained faithful to forensic medicine and emergency medicine and continue to be convinced that both subjects have many more interfaces than is commonly expected. The additional knowledge from forensic medicine can broaden emergency medical horizons, facilitate decisions and make backgrounds plausible. However, not only we but also medicine itself has developed further in the last 10 years, so that in this new edition not only figures have been updated, but we have also dealt intensively once again with all the contents. We have supplemented, expanded and updated them. In particular, the chapter on child abuse has increased significantly in scope. This topic is very close to our hearts and we hope that the assistance we provide there will be of practical use.

With Springer Verlag we have also found a new publisher for our paperback who also believes that the synergies from emergency medicine and forensic medicine should be used. Many thanks to the trust placed in us, especially to Dr. Krätz and Mr. Treiber, who supported us from the publishing side.

Our thanks also go to our families. Our three children know that for us, work is not just a task, but a passion, and they accept when mum is on her mobile phone or dad has to rush from playing to an emergency. We are very happy and know that it is not a matter of course for Prof. Dr. Michael Bohnert to continue to support us and the project in addition to his work as Director of the Institute of Forensic Medicine at the University Hospital of Würzburg. Without him, this new edition would simply not have come about in this quality.

Horben, Germany
Summer 2020

Sieglinde Ahne
Thomas Ahne

Preface and Introduction to the First Edition

There had never been so many "aha-experiences" in the course of medical studies as in the unfortunately very short block practical course in forensic medicine. We constantly remembered situations from our former full-time, now part-time work in the rescue service, in which we would have made different decisions or taken or omitted measures with basic knowledge of forensic medicine. It quickly became clear that it was not just us who felt this way, but that it is widespread in emergency medicine to know little or nothing about the work of forensic medicine. Everyone is familiar with the relevant TV series and in quite a few films the forensic doctor virtually pushes the emergency doctor aside at the scene of the incident – this probably has nothing to do with real life. In reality, however, there are a surprisingly large number of points of contact between the two specialties, but one rarely notices this in the rescue service, since in practice the fields are usually deployed one after the other without meeting in person. Due to ignorance, many possible synergies for both fields remain unused. Prof. Bohnert was quickly convinced that this grievance had to be tackled jointly. In the following, Prof. Bohnert represented the side of forensic medicine, we represented the side of emergency medicine, and so we were able to compile the facts of forensic medicine relevant to emergency medicine in a constructive dialogue – without Prof. Bohnert's indispensable expertise, the book would simply not have been possible. Many thanks for this! The idea of a practical guide was quickly born, because in this way it is possible to address many interested people in addition to further training events and the reader can call up the facts again at any time. Certainly, the present book will be carried in the pocket of only a few, but we have deliberately set the size to a paperback format, because we did not want to create a new textbook on legal medicine, but a book tailored for emergency medicine practitioners with the details relevant to this group of people, in addition, the text should be short and concise, because the training time is known to be scarce, especially in health care, and not infrequently extends to the personal and bitterly fought for free time.

We were very pleased that we promptly succeeded in inspiring Thieme Verlag with our idea; Mrs Engeli, Mrs Heuser as well as Mrs Addicks supported us tirelessly in the realisation of the project. Of course, we would also like to thank our families, who supported us during the preparation of the manuscript. Also thanks to our daughter Alexa, who was born during this time, because she patiently endured countless hours next to our desks and had to listen to many discussions regarding the text drafts and our mind games.

It is our sincere hope that this practical guide can contribute noticeably in daily work, not least in the reader's own interest, to act in a legally sound manner and to recognise and promote the points of intersection between emergency and forensic medicine, so that in future these commonalities can be used more effectively. This book is intended to appeal to all those working in emergency medicine, whether from a medical or non-medical background; for simplicity, the term doctor has often been used in the text. However, we are aware that a large number of patients in the German emergency medical services are not seen by a doctor at all in the prehospital setting, so the same standards are to be applied in principle to non-medical emergency medical services personnel as to doctors. Only the legal requirements for medical staff are often stricter, but the competences are broader (e.g. necropsy). Likewise, we understand it as a matter of course that female employees in the rescue service are addressed in the same way as the male colleagues named in the text.

We are very grateful for constructive criticism from the readership, as it contributes to the further development of this project.

Horben, Germany Thomas Ahne
Spring 2010 Sieglinde Ahne

Contents

About the Authors

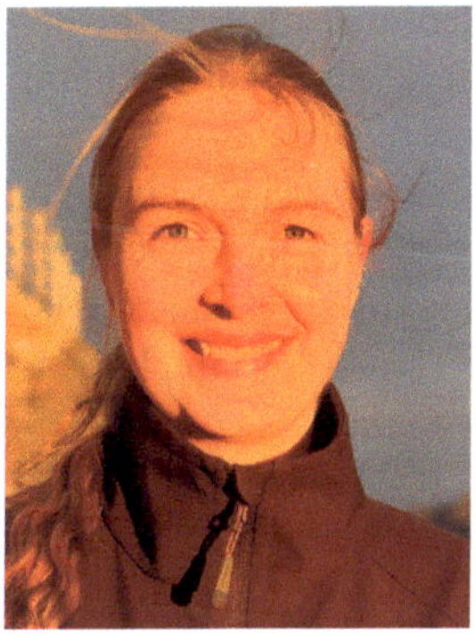

Sieglinde Ahne med. state examination 2012 since 2014 at the Institute of Forensic Medicine of the Albert-Ludwigs-University Freiburg as assistant physician 2014–2015 Creation of an e-learning program for physicians and students on the topic of child abuse for the Competence Center Child Protection in Medicine Baden-Württemberg (Com.can) 2015–2017 Collaboration in the creation of the e-learning program "Basic Course Child Protection in Medicine" under the direction of Prof. Dr. J.M. Fegert/Ulm Since 2017, working as a consultant at the medical child protection hotline Mother of three children (4, 7, 11)

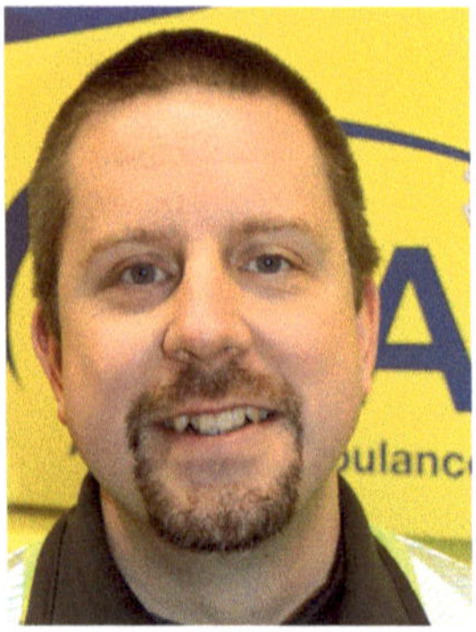

Thomas Ahne Born in 1980, initially a teaching assistant and organisational head of rescue services as well as ERC instructor. Studied human medicine in Freiburg, 2010–2016 residency in anaesthesiology at the University Hospital Freiburg. Subsequently worked at the Clinic for Anesthesiology at the Loretto Hospital Freiburg and in the Internal Intensive Care Medicine of the University Hospital Freiburg. Since 2019, lateral entry into general medicine at the Todtnau Health Centre.

Active ground and air-bound emergency physician in Germany and Switzerland. Medical director of the emergency service DRK Lörrach and school doctor of the educational institution Bad Säckingen of the DRK Landesschule Baden-Württemberg.

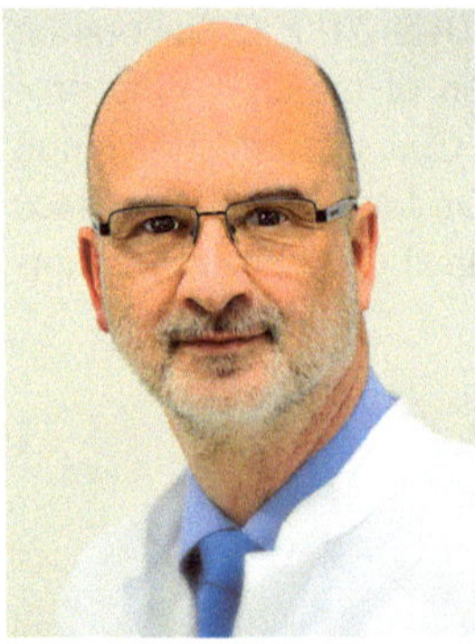

Michael Bohnert Studied human medicine 1985–1992 in Freiburg. Further training in forensic medicine at the Institute of Pathology of the Constance Hospitals, at the Psychiatric University Hospital of Freiburg, at the Institute of Forensic Medicine of the University of Bern and at the Institute of Forensic Medicine of the University Hospital of Freiburg. Habilitation in Forensic Medicine in 2001 at the University of Freiburg. Since 2010 Director of the Institute of Legal Medicine at the University of Würzburg.

1 Links Between Emergency and Forensic Medicine

During the practical work in the rescue service on the one hand and the medical work in forensic medicine on the other hand, it becomes clear again and again that it is widespread in emergency medicine to know nothing or only little about the work of forensic medicine. Everyone knows the relevant TV series and in quite a few movies the forensic doctor practically pushes the emergency doctor aside at the scene of the emergency – but this probably has nothing to do with real life. In reality, however, there are a surprisingly large number of points of contact between the two specialties, of which one rarely notices anything in the emergency medical services, because in practice the individual areas are usually deployed one after the other without meeting in person. Thus, many possible synergies for both fields often remain unused.

The idea of a practical guide was quickly born, because it can be used as a supplement to training events to address many interested parties, and the facts can be called up again for the reader at any time.

Certainly, the present book will be carried in the pocket of only a few, but we have deliberately set the size to a paperback format, because we did not want to create a new textbook on legal medicine, but a book tailored for emergency medicine practitioners with the details relevant to this group of people. In addition, the text had to be short and concise in each case, as it is well known that training time is scarce, especially in the healthcare sector, and

S. Ahne et al., *Forensic aspects in emergency medicine*,
https://doi.org/10.1007/978-3-662-65949-6_1

not infrequently extends to personal and bitterly fought-for free time.

This book is intended to address all those involved in emergency medicine, whether doctor or paramedic; for simplicity, the term physician has often been used in the text. However, we are aware that a large number of patients in the German emergency medical services are not seen by a physician in the prehospital setting; therefore, the same standards are to be applied in principle to nonphysician emergency medical services personel as to physicians. Only the legal requirements for medical staff are often stricter, but the competences are broader (e.g. the external examination of the body). We also understand it as a matter of course that female employees in the rescue service are addressed here in the same way as their male colleagues named in the text.

Absolute practical relevance was the premise for each chapter of this book. There are enough textbooks of forensic medicine, but they do not illuminate the interface with emergency medicine. Our aim is to fill this gap. It does not matter to emergency medical services personel how exactly molecular genetic detection methods work or what species of fly populates the corpse at what time in a particular region, although it is not uncommon for us to be led to believe this in public. Rather, it is of almost daily importance in emergency medicine to be able to assess, for example, the significance of injuries and the threat they may pose to the patient. It is one of the last services rendered to a human being to perform a sufficient postmortem examination and determine what the manner of death is in any given case. Again and again investigations show that also in Germany the quality of the corpse inspection often leaves much to be desired. This new edition begins in the same way as a patient is encountered in the field – first the behavior at the alleged crime scene, then the documentation and then the more precise theory behind the various intersections of the two sectors forensic medicine and emergency medicine.

2 Behaviour at the Scene

2.1 Casuistry

On a hot August afternoon you are called to a middle-class residential area under the keyword "unconscious person". When you arrive at the address, you are greeted by a neighbour who states that he has found his 84-year-old neighbour, who lives alone, lifeless in the apartment. He had gained access to the flat by means of the key deposited with him for emergencies, after the neighbour did not open the door when she heard music coming from the flat.

You find an unclothed woman lying on the floor in the kitchen area of the ground-floor apartment who shows certain signs of death (lividity, rigor mortis). Since you cannot rule out an unnatural cause of death and the situation in which the body is found seems strange to you, you confine yourself to the pure determination of death without a post-mortem examination and inform the police. After approx. 15 min, a patrol car crew arrives, to whom you briefly explain the circumstances before a new operation takes you away from the scene.

About 3 h later, the criminal investigation department calls with the following questions:

S. Ahne et al., *Forensic aspects in emergency medicine*,
https://doi.org/10.1007/978-3-662-65949-6_2

- Was the patio door already open?
- The appearance of the hypostasis suggests that there must have been a repositioning after death. Was the body moved by the rescue service?
- Did you tell the neighbour that Mrs. X had died of a heart attack?
- You can see a hematoma in the left inside of the elbow, was there a puncture attempt by the paramedics?

Only after consultation with the entire rescue service team can the situation and the activities/measures carried out be determined to some extent. After a longer protocol recording at the police station, you are annoyed about the high expenditure of time for this operation and ask yourself what could be done better in such a situation.

2.2 Introduction

Fortunately, only a minority of rescue service operations involve a criminal offence. Nevertheless, by providing "on-site assistance", it is not uncommon to arrive at the scene of a criminally relevant matter. In doing so, it is very important to act professionally, objectively and purposefully by fulfilling one's acute medical mission. However, one should try to keep a keen eye on the locality while in the field. This can be relevant for a later reconstruction of the event, a better assessment of the accident kinetics or for inquiries by the investigating authorities. A further aim should be to change the existing trace situation only as little as absolutely necessary, even if emergency medical measures have priority over securing evidence in any case. All observations and findings should be adequately documented, even if this means an increased expenditure of time; it could later be an important aspect in legal proceedings.

2.3 Basic Rules

In principle, there are few, but nevertheless very important basic rules for the emergency medical technician to follow at the scene of the accident:

2.3.1 Saving Life Before Securing Evidence

As long as there is only the slightest suspicion that death has not yet occurred irreversibly, life-saving measures must be taken. As banal as this sounds, in the case of (seemingly) obvious violent crimes one tends to wait hesitantly at first because one is afraid of doing something wrong; however, every moment of waiting is too long. There is no difference between this and other calls for service. The police, prosecutor, or forensic pathologist cannot blame the rescue team if the finding situation is altered in order to take emergency medical action. Clearly, the spatial situation must be altered to gain better access to the patient, and in some circumstances the patient may even be transported to a hospital without first being seen by an investigating officer. A delay in medical treatment is not tolerable.

2.3.2 The Whodunit in the Head

Part of being a professional in acute care is relying only on facts. Nevertheless, it is all too easy for an alleged offence to give rise to suspicions that cannot be proven. As the name implies, investigative authorities are responsible for locating a perpetrator, if indeed there is one, and initiating criminal proceedings. The emergency medical team is only a (rather involuntary) witness to the event and has a purely descriptive function. There should be no private detectives in red jackets!

Nevertheless, the rescue team has an important role to play: it is not uncommon for the rescue service to have the first contact with the person concerned, and no one later sees the spatial arrangements as they were in the finding situation – there are actually always (unintentional) changes in the spatial situation. Everyone in the team, from the trainee to the experienced emergency doctor, has the duty to note conspicuities as precisely as possible and to inform the investigating authorities of them. However, it is sometimes not so easy to separate exactly what one has observed objectively and what is already subject to a personal interpretation. Example: A man is lying lifeless with obviously serious injuries in front of a high-rise building, a cleaning cloth is lying next to him and the window on the sixth floor is open. These are precisely the facts; the fact that he may have fallen out of the window while cleaning it must be the subject of objective investigation by the police, even if this cause initially suggests itself. Another example is shown in Fig. 2.1.

Each of us is influenced by the countless descriptions of crime, whether as a book, a film or in the newspaper, and it is precisely for this reason that we find it difficult only to describe and not to interpret.

2.3.3 Definition of Location/Crime Scene

The title of this chapter speaks of the crime scene, but one should always include in one's considerations that the place of discovery need not be the same as the crime scene. There may be no evidence or only discrete evidence of a discrepancy between the two locations, it is not always the infamous dead diver in the woods. Factually, there is often no definitive proof that the event took place at the eventual location where it was found. It is not uncommon in capital crimes for the victim to be moved to another location or position after the crime in order to cover up existing traces, to lay new ones, or to feign a different factual situation (so-called body dumping, Figs. 2.2 and 2.3). It may also have been the intention of the perpetrator to bring the victim to exactly this place.

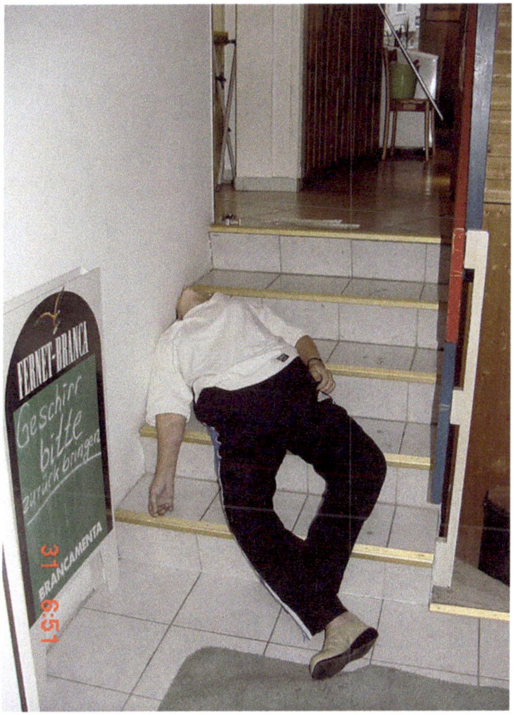

Fig. 2.1 Misleading finding of a natural death from myocardial infarction at the workplace. The death was not the result of a fall down stairs, but the fall was the result of circulatory failure

2.3.4 Collection of Information

If irreversible death has definitely occurred and an unnatural cause of death is obvious, it is advisable for all those involved to withdraw and to await the arrival of the police. During this time, no further search for information should take place; for example, searching for old doctor's notes in the files in the living room cupboard is not appropriate and is not the task of the rescue service. Instead, care must be taken to ensure that no more people are put in the position of having to change any traces. Likewise, information must only be passed on to authorised persons, namely the

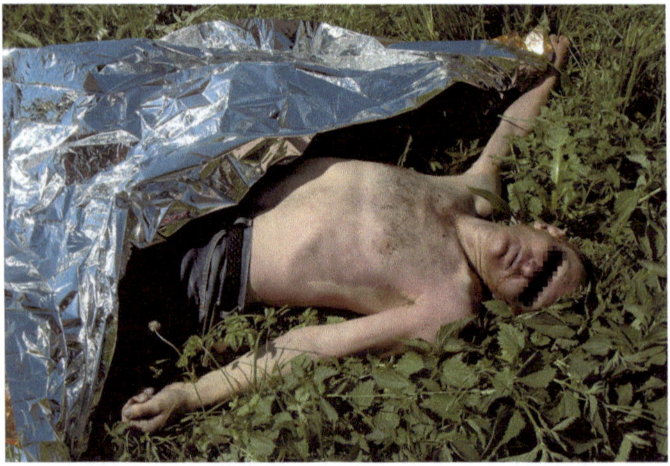

Fig. 2.2 Drugged corpse deposited at the site some time after death. This is supported by the following findings: The position and distribution of the death marks do not match the supine position in which the corpse was found

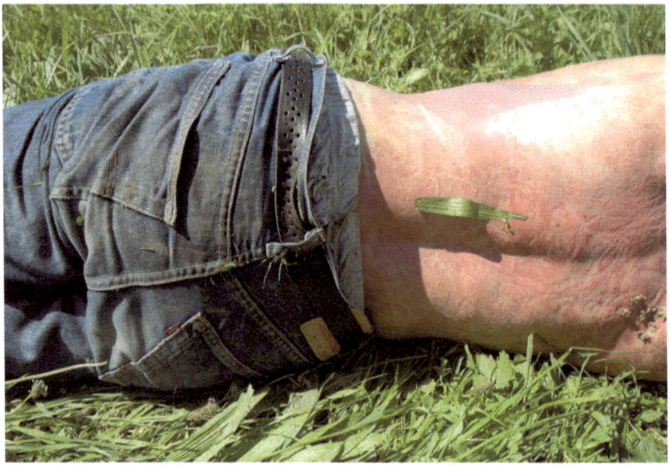

Fig. 2.3 Clear abrasion marks can be seen on the back waistband of the trousers

police. Information to other persons is to be strictly refrained from, here the general duty of confidentiality is of particular importance.

The following aids to action can be identified:

- Look, grasp, be silent
- Stop at the door frame
- gather impressions
- Pay attention to the little things
- At first appearances we must be suspicious
- No rash movements
- Hands in the pockets
- Keep your mouth shut – no giving out information to unauthorized people (anyone but the police).
- Do not reconstruct too early
- Try to remember all the changes that have already been made and the original location, making notes and sketches if necessary.

2.3.5 Photo Documentation

Any photo documentation of the detection situation and the following measures is a double-edged sword. On the one hand, it is an excellent opportunity to record the situation almost perfectly true to the original (Fig. 2.4); on the other hand, it must not violate applicable law and ethical boundaries must be maintained. In any case, all photographic material must be handed over to the police and subsequently all data must be deleted. As is well known, it is not permitted to photograph people without their consent; this also applies to deceased persons. In general, but especially in the case of an investigation, photographic material may not be passed on or used at one's own discretion – an ongoing investigation prohibits the further use of the photographic material. After the end of the proceedings, this is also only possible with alienation of the person in accordance with the usual requirements of personality protection, for example in the context of training events. It is more

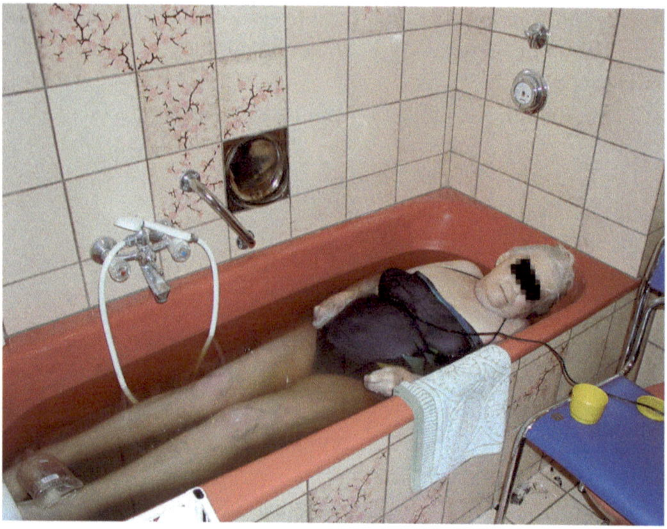

Fig. 2.4 Typical location of suicide by electrocution in the bathtub

than advisable to delete image material in one's own possession before it is used incorrectly.

2.4 Behaviour Towards ...

2.4.1 ... The Victim

If the victim of a physical assault is responsive, he or she should be met with maximum empathy and a professional demeanor. A calm, level-headed manner with a stringent goal in action is the key to success. The victim may be in an emotionally catastrophic situation with seemingly no way out. Comforting physical contact must be established; this is a great help to some patients, others are less able to deal with it. Psychosocial care should be considered at an early stage. Of course, somatic treatment is the first priority.

Nevertheless, a neutral behaviour is indicated and the injured party must not be influenced in his opinion. Of course, the police should be encouraged to investigate the incident – in the case of serious offences, the police should be informed anyway, because then there is an interest in investigation even without a direct order from the injured party. Sometimes there is no sharp distinction between the roles of victim and perpetrator, but an assessment of this is not the task of emergency medicine.

All emergency medical measures must be accurately documented so that they can be distinguished from other physical changes in retrospect. For example, all unsuccessful puncture attempts must also be documented so that the puncture sites are not considered to be older puncture sites. If the injured person dies during the course of care, all medical supplies must be left on the deceased.

2.4.2 ... The Relatives

On the part of the victim's relatives, there is understandably a great need for information. Even if this is understandable, the duty of confidentiality must nevertheless be observed; with the authorization of the injured party, all medical findings may of course be passed on. If this explicit authorization cannot be obtained, the probable will of the patient is decisive. In case of doubt, one should only very briefly mention the medical condition and refer to later detailed information by the injured party himself or by the investigating authorities. Here, too, it is not always clear to what extent third parties were and are involved in the event, so one must be cautious about passing on information. Psychosocial support may also need to be organised short for the relatives.

2.4.3 ... The Offender

Possible physical injuries or other health impairments (e.g. drug influence) of the perpetrator must also be determined and treated immediately. Even if it is sometimes difficult, a professional appearance is also required here. When taking the case history, one should concentrate only on the physical condition and not on the course of events, despite all personal interests. Influencing the perpetrator to make any statements is of course forbidden. As already indicated, it must also be stressed here that an alleged perpetrator can also be a victim in some way and needs help.

2.4.4 ... The Investigating Authorities

Cooperation between the rescue service and the police usually works well. The more serious an offence is, the more professional the cooperation must be. It is important that the rescue team concentrates on its original tasks and additionally only records the observations made without any interpretation. It has to be reminded again that the emergency medical therapy of the patient has priority over investigative activities. Especially if, due to these measures, no parallel questioning of the involved persons by the police is possible, questioning/information gathering must not be carried out by the rescue team, as otherwise one has to accept the accusation of influencing. Good documentation of the events and observations made is important, so that adequate information on the facts can be given to the police even after a long delay. As a rule, it will be necessary for the police to carry out extensive questioning outside of regular working hours, as concentration and therefore also the ability to remember things will suffer during the required readiness for action.

Any necessary changes to the place of discovery must be reported to the investigating authorities so that this does not result in a different trace picture.

2.4.5 ... The Press/Public

As a rule, it is not appropriate to release information to the public, possibly via the press. In the event of increased media interest, all larger institutions in the rescue sector should appoint a press spokesperson who has also been trained accordingly and therefore knows exactly what information may be published and what requires secrecy in terms of confidentiality. Film recordings in particular should be viewed critically, as the right to one's own image is easily violated here, both on the patient side and on the side of the rescuer.

2.4.6 Special Case of a Helper as a Defendant

Should the situation arise that a helper (regardless of qualification) is accused of a physical offence against the patient, it must be ensured immediately that treatment by new staff is adequate and prompt. Police should be called in early, preferably before the situation escalates, to document the facts expeditiously. Detailed documentation is essential and appropriate superiors must be informed.

2.4.7 Helpers as Victims

Unfortunately, it is becoming more and more common for helpers to be attacked by patients, relatives, but also by uninvolved third parties, both verbally and physically. Year after year, there is an increasing number of attacks against rescue personnel. Self-protection is the top priority! Even if it is difficult, one should try not to let oneself be provoked by verbal attacks, but rather withdraw as quickly as possible with the patient, for example into the ambulance. The principles of tactical medicine, which actually originate from the military context, can also come into play here. This does not involve the use of force against aggressors, but rather self-protection and de-escalation. Even an active act in self-defence should only be the last resort in individual cases. Fortunately, the legislator has also recognized this increasing and serious problem and has increased the penalties accordingly. There are already rescue services that equip their employees with bulletproof or stab-proof vests. Modern vests are not very bulky and can be worn concealed. The open wearing of leather gloves, pepper spray or other defensive weapons is to be seen very critically because of their potentially provocative effect.

Documentation of Injuries 3

Medical care of injured persons has priority over forensic documentation of findings. However, one does not exclude the other and the documentation of injuries can certainly be integrated into wound treatment. Above all, it is essential to realise that not only the clinical but also the forensic view of an injured person is important. From the emergency physician's point of view, the focus is primarily on injuries that have therapeutic and prognostic relevance, i.e. that require treatment. In contrast, injuries that do not require treatment, such as haematomas, tend to be neglected. Although they are noticed, they are given secondary consideration and – as experience has shown – are often only mentioned in italics in the documentation of findings or are sometimes even forgotten. From a forensic point of view, however, injuries that have no therapeutic consequences are also relevant, as they also allow conclusions to be drawn about the course of events.

The form of an injury can be used to draw conclusions about the type of force involved (for details, see Chap. 5). The anatomical localization and distribution of the injuries provide clues as to how the injury occurred, in particular as to whether it was an accident, inflicted by a third party or self-inflicted.

The assessment of bleeding injuries on site and in poor lighting is inherently flawed, but it is nevertheless useful to document the wound by taking photographs before treatment. No sophisticated camera equipment is necessary for this – photos can be taken with

S. Ahne et al., *Forensic aspects in emergency medicine*,
https://doi.org/10.1007/978-3-662-65949-6_3

any smartphone, which can help in the forensic medical assessment at a later date. Any photo is better than no photo. Even better, however, are photos that can be used to attribute the findings afterwards. To do this, a few basic principles must be observed:

- Portrait, make overviews for the identifiability of the person taken. This is also possible as a snapshot during the care incidentally. The images should show the person, not just detailed findings.
- Partial overviews with anatomical landmarks help to clearly locate injuries on the body on the images and to estimate size ratios.
- Details are best photographed with scale or at least in such a way that the size can be estimated from anatomical structures on the photographs (e.g. Figs. 3.1 and 3.2).
- Pay attention to focus, color, completeness, lighting, angle. Be careful when using the flash: Often the essential findings are over-illuminated and the images are not true to color.
- Always save photos as originals.
- Save metadata (recording date, recording time, possibly recording location).

Whether and to what extent such photo documentation will be relevant for investigation cannot be foreseen at the time of deployment. However, it is important that they are taken and that the existence of the photographs is made known to the police. In addition to such photos, documentation sheets can also be used. Although these are generally not intended for use on site, but rather for examination in an ambulance, they can be used as a checklist to help ensure that no potentially important forensic findings are overlooked or forgotten after the operation. "Injuries" resulting from medical procedures must be documented in the incident log. They can cause confusion afterwards if their genesis is not clear (see Chap. 8).

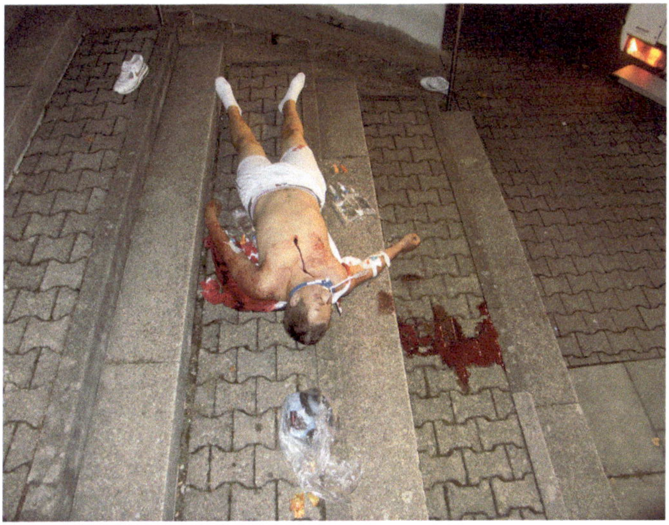

Fig. 3.1 Homicide by singular stab to the heart. Finding situation after attempted resuscitation by the emergency physician

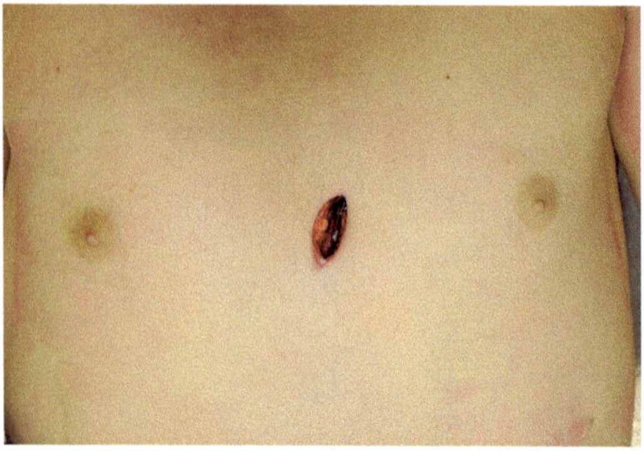

Fig. 3.2 Detail of stab wound with clear physical reference points

4 Thanatology

Thanatology is literally translated the study of death. It refers to all the processes that take place in the human body during dying and after death. The findings are used in the medical post-mortem examination to determine death, and some can also be used to narrow down the time of death.

Dying is a process, even in those cases where death occurs very quickly. The phase from the beginning of the dying process is called agony (translated: death throes). It can be very short, for example in the case of a death within seconds due to cardiac arrhythmia, but it can also last for many hours, for example in the final phase of a tumour disease. In some cases it can be interrupted by resuscitation measures, and in the best case (if resuscitation is successful) it can also be terminated. Agony leads to clinical death, which is characterized by cardiovascular arrest and respiratory failure. This is potentially reversible by cardiopulmonary resuscitation. If no resuscitation measures are taken or they are unsuccessful, then individual death follows after a few minutes. This is considered to be an irreversible failure of the brain and the whole organism.

The brain is the organ that is affected earliest by circulatory arrest, as it has a resuscitation time of only about 8 min under normal conditions. In hypothermia, this can be significantly prolonged. Brain death is equated with individual death. The resuscitation time of other organs is much longer (e.g. heart up to 30 min,

S. Ahne et al., *Forensic aspects in emergency medicine*,
https://doi.org/10.1007/978-3-662-65949-6_4

Table 4.1 AEIOU rule – reasons for apparent death

A	Anemia, alcohol
E	Electric current
I	Injury (especially craniocerebral trauma)
O	Opium (representing narcotics or psychotropic drugs)
U	Uremia (representative of metabolic coma), hypothermia

kidney up to 2 h). Independent of this is the ability of various cells and tissues to show limited responses to external stimuli, which is referred to as supravitality. One example is the ability of skeletal muscles to contract in response to a mechanical or electrical stimulus, which is used as a parameter in forensic medicine to determine the time of death.

In agony as well as in the phase of clinical death, the body appears lifeless and the person may be mistaken for dead. Uncertain signs of death may be: pulselessness, no measurable blood pressure, no visible cardiac activity in the ECG, breathlessness, decreased body temperature, no peripheral reflexes, no defensive reactions to pain stimuli, dilated pupils. None of these signs, nor the combination of several signs, should tempt one to assume and document the death of a person. For this condition there is the term "apparent death", also called vita minima or vita reducta. In fact, numerous pathological or traumatic reasons exist for this, such as hypothermia, metabolic crisis, traumatic brain injury, or intoxication. As a mnemonic, there is the AEIOU rule, in which reasons for the presence of a vita minima are assigned to each vowel (Table 4.1).

4.1 Early Signs of Death

The earliest sure sign of death is the postmortem hypostasis also known as livor morits. They appear about 20 min after circulatory arrest, i.e. at a time when the brain's resuscitation time is far exceeded. The first hypostasis are easy to overlook, because they are single, spotted reddenings of the skin. Only as they progress do they become extensive and confluent. Livor mortis are caused by blood that is no longer circulating, sinking passively into the dependent parts of the body due to gravity, which ultimately leads to blood filling the skin capillaries, which becomes visible as a blue-violet discoloration of the skin (Fig. 4.1). This colour, known as "livid", is a consequence of the O_2 depletion of the red blood cells; the oxygen saturation of the blood in the hypostasis is at most a few percent. A bright red discoloration of the livor mortis may be the result of reoxygenation of the red blood cells, as occurs with several hours of postmortem cold exposure (Fig. 4.2). However, it may also be a consequence of CO intoxication. In particular,cherry-red staining of the hypostasis throughout, including under the fingernails or toenails, on the palms of the hands or soles of the feet, should be recognised at post-mortem examination as a sign of CO poisoning. In cold-induced bright red hypostasis, these are usually "zoned," meaning that blue-violet color components are also found, especially next to the contact areas, which are recessed from the hypostasis. Recesses of the hypostasis are found everywhere on the body, where a counter-pressure from the outside prevented a filling of the skin capillar-

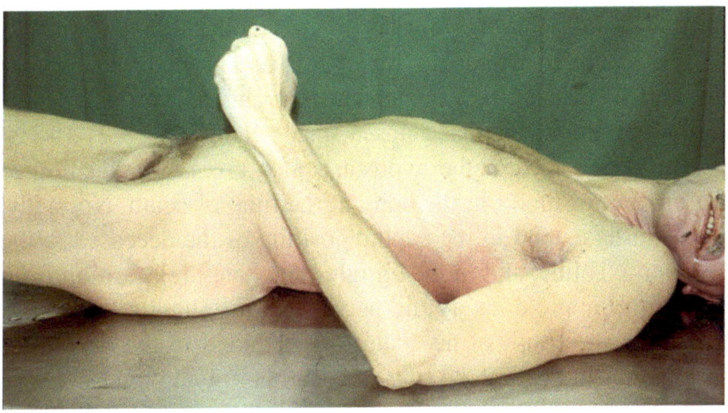

Fig. 4.1 Typical distribution of livor mortis for the supine position. Rigor mortis has occurred in the flexed position of the elbow

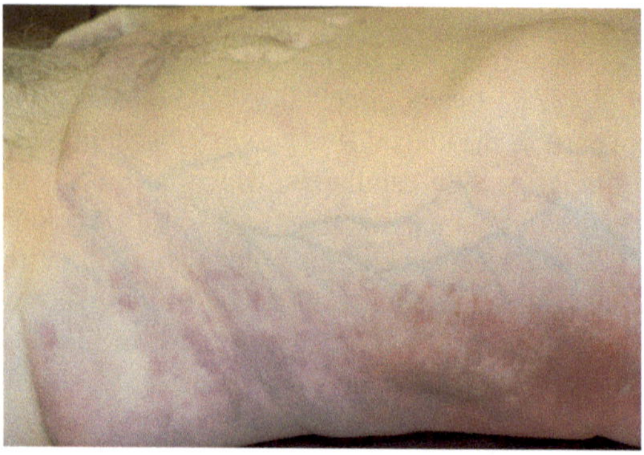

Fig. 4.2 Zoned hypostasis on the lateral part of the trunk. In the lower part livid stained, in the upper part light red staining due to postmortem cold exposure

Table 4.2 Hypostasis over time

Start	15–20 min
Confluence	0.5–2 h
Complete relocatability	2–6 h
Incomplete transferability	4–24 h
Complete push away capability	1–20 h

ies, i.e. beside the contact areas also there, where close-fitting parts of clothing or other objects pressed on the body.

The extent to which the hypostasis are pronounced, wether they can be pushed away and can be rearranged, gives some indication of the time that has elapsed since death (Table 4.2).

The appearance of the hypostasis also gives an indication of the amount of blood in the body at the time of death. Normally, livor mortis extend in the supine position of the deceased to the anterior axis line, and in the upright (e.g. hanging) position from the feet to approximately the pelvic region. Slightly hypostasis are either the result of an acute loss of blood to the outside or inside, thus indicating the cause of death, or of chronic anaemia.

The second sure sign of death, which follows somewhat later in time, is rigor mortis (see Fig. 4.1). It is caused by the acampsia

Table 4.3 Time course of rigor mortis under non-cooled conditions

Muscle relaxation	Immediately
Onset of rigor mortis	0.5–7 h
Reversion to rigidity	<20 h
Maximum rigidity	2–20 h
Complete solution of rigidity	>24 h

of the musculature and thus of the joints due to the successive drop in ATP levels in the musculature. Rigidity begins at the earliest half an hour after the onset of death, whereby this time depends on the pre-mortem muscle activity and thus the ATP content: muscles that were already heavily used during life become rigid more quickly than muscles that were at rest and therefore have full ATP stores. For this reason, the order in which individual muscle groups become rigid is highly variable. In the first, according to recent studies up to 20 h after death, rigor mortis may reappear if it has been broken. When fully developed, rigor mortis is difficult to break in the large joints of a muscular body. In the course of the following days it resolves itself, which is the result of proteolysis due to putrefaction, a process which occurs more rapidly the higher the ambient temperature. The time course of the onset and resolution of rigor mortis is temperature dependent. Cold slows down the times listed in the table (see Table 4.3).

4.2 Late Signs of Death

Late signs of death are decay, often associated with animal feeding in the warm season (Fig. 4.3), putrefaction, mummification, corpse lipid formation or tanning. Putrefaction, animal feeding and decay lead to skeletonization, whereas mummification, corpse lipid formation or tanning lead to some preservation of soft tissues. The occurrence of the various forms depends on the environmental conditions. The most common in Germany is putrefaction.

Putrefaction is the result of bacterial colonization of the corpse by endogenous, predominantly anaerobic germs from the intestinal tract. For this reason, the first signs of putrefaction are usually

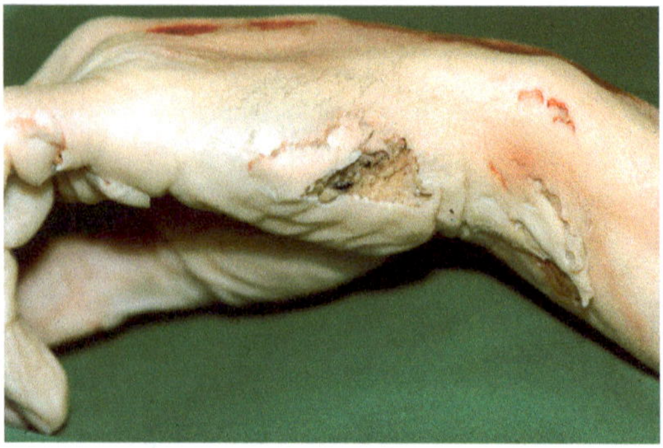

Fig. 4.3 Skin defects on the hand and forearm with characteristic jagged to arcuate borders, without accompanying hemorrhages of the soft tissues: post-mortem animal feeding by rodents

found on the abdominal skin and here in the right lower abdomen. This is a green discoloration of the skin (Fig. 4.4), which is subsequently joined by a vesicular detachment of the epidermis, gas inflation of the soft tissues, leakage of fluid from the respiratory orifices, penetration of the vein markings on the skin (Fig. 4.5) and, over time, detachment of the epidermis (Fig. 4.6). The development of the decay findings proceeds in certain sequences, depending on temperature (Table 4.4). A characteristic feature is also the foul, sweet odor, which is caused by the decomposition of musculature and other soft tissue. It is – in addition to the rather unattractive appearance – an important reason why people do not like to deal with dead bodies so closely during post-mortem examinations if they are rotten. This instinctive reluctance often leads to less care being taken in the post-mortem examination than is the case with "fresh" corpses. It is important to realize this. Furthermore, it is important to know that decomposed corpses are not automatically considered infectious; in fact, the risk of becoming infected during post-mortem examinations is considered very low, even in the case of those who have died of infectious diseases, if basic hygiene measures are observed. Most importantly, however, it is important to know that death per se is not infectious and that there is no such thing as "corpse poison".

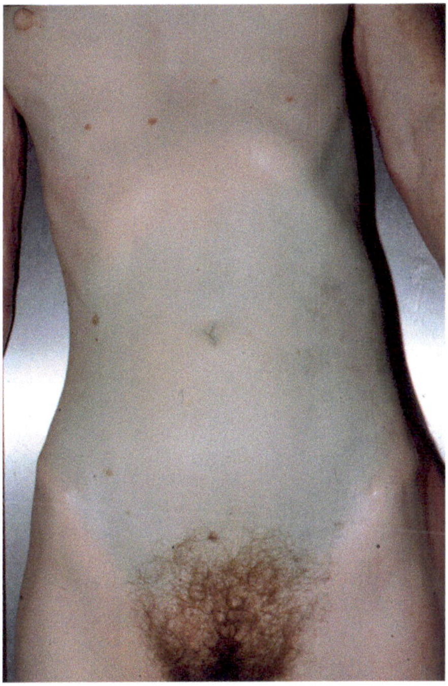

Fig. 4.4 Beginning of rot: green discoloration of abdominal skin

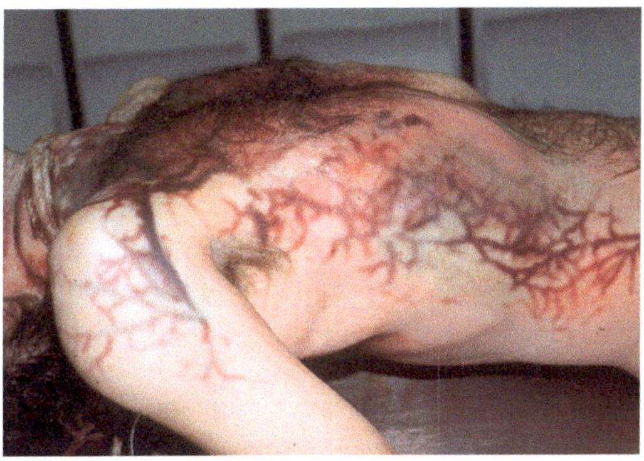

Fig. 4.5 Penetration of the venous net on the torso of a hanged person

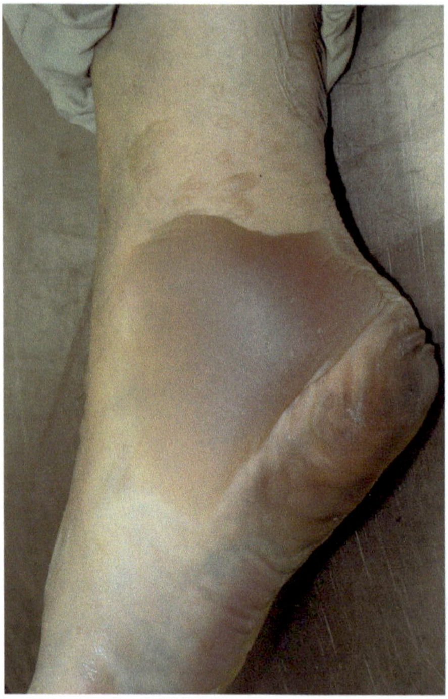

Fig. 4.6 Decay: blistered detachment of the epidermis on the ankle

Especially in the warm season, rot is often combined with an infestation by fly maggots. The laying of eggs by the female flies can already take place in the agony phase, the infestation by fly maggots is not a sure sign of death! However, it is an indication of dead tissue – fly maggots only eat this, not vital tissue, which is why they can also be used in necrosis ablation on the living patient. In the deceased, oviposition occurs as soon as temperatures are above 10 °C and it is light (Fig. 4.7). Preferably, the egg clusters are deposited in the eye clefts, the respiratory orifices, the external auditory canals, the genital region, moist macerated skin folds or wounds, as the fly maggots have the best starting conditions here (Fig. 4.8). The growth of fly maggots is about 1–1.5 mm per day, the whole development cycle with pupation and hatching

Table 4.4 Time course of decay changes of a body

1–2 days	Greenish discoloration of the abdominal skin Softening of the eyeballs
3–7 days	Spread of green putrefaction Penetration of the venous networks Discharge of putrefactive liquid from the respiratory openings Skin rot blisters
8–12 days	Surface discolouration of the body surface Surface detachment of the epidermis Gas bloating of the abdomen, darkening of the face Hair extensible
14–21 days	Strong gas inflation of the body Sunken eyes Nails extendable Beginning secondary mummification

of the next generation of adult flies about 14 days. Therefore, if there are no empty pupal barrels yet to be found on the corpse, then (assuming rapid oviposition after death) death should not have been more than 2 weeks ago.

The term "putrefaction" is often used as an umbrella term for post-mortem corpse decomposition, but this is not correct. Putrefaction is a specific form of corpse decomposition in which mainly aerobic bacteria play a role. Putrefaction occurs primarily in cool (and somewhat moist) environmental conditions, such as those found in crypts or outdoors during the cold season. There are, however, many mixed pictures between putrefaction and decomposition; a differentiated distinction between the two forms of decomposition is not of importance in rescue service practice.

A finding frequently encountered at least on ears, nose, hands and feet at the onset of later corpse symptoms is mummification, i.e. the drying out of tissue, which then turns brownish to blackish, shrinks and can become firm like rind (Fig. 4.9). The coexistence of rot, maggot feeding and desiccation on the same corpse is not uncommon. Since progressive putrefaction leads to a depletion of the corpse's fluids and the growth conditions for the bacteria thus become increasingly poor, it is not uncommon for mummification to occur in putrefied corpses, a process known as secondary mummification; this is then a dried fixed image of the

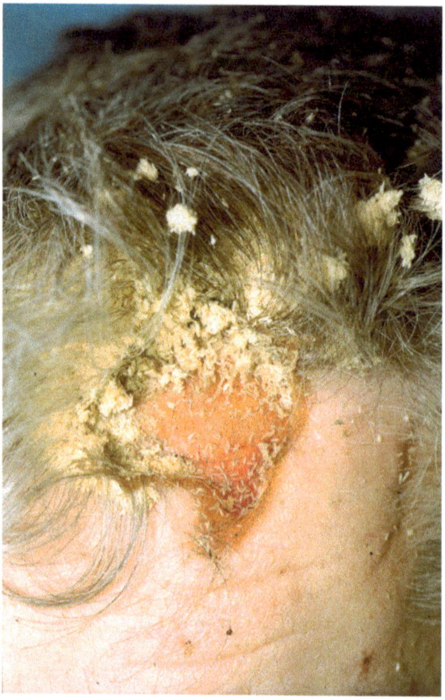

Fig. 4.7 Numerous fly eggs next to a skin defect at the forehead-hair interface

state of putrefaction previously reached. Such state images can remain stable for a very long time, as is reported again and again with so-called apartment corpses, which are sometimes found only after months or even years.

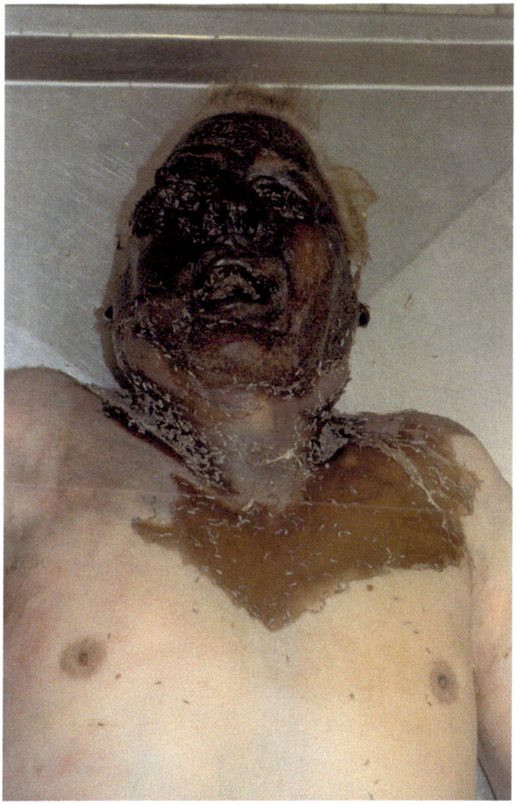

Fig. 4.8 Post-mortem infestation with fly maggots on the head, neck and upper thorax. The black discoloration of the skin is a consequence of the digestive enzymes secreted by the maggots

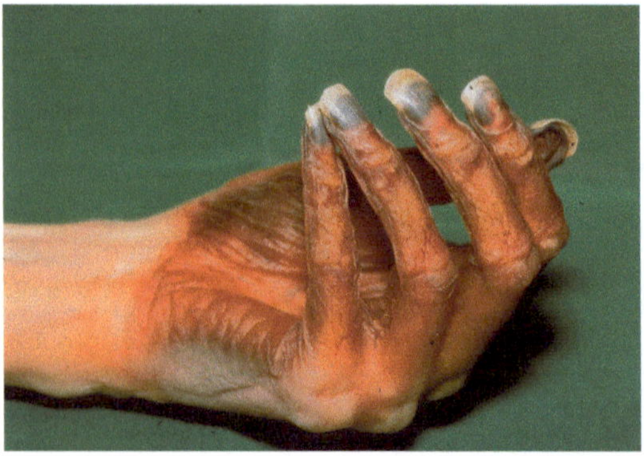

Fig. 4.9 Mummification of the hand: drying and shrinkage of skin and soft tissues

5 Forensic Traumatology

5.1 General

Traumatology is the study of injuries. Forensic traumatology deals with the various forms of violence and their reconstructive aspects. This includes on the one hand the recognition of the type of violence from the wound findings, on the other hand the assessment of the type of origin (accident, externally inflicted, self-inflicted), the vitality of a finding, the age of an injury and the dangerousness of an injury.

In the case of violence, a distinction is made between the forms:

- Blunt force
- Semi sharp force
- Sharp force
- Projectiles
- Abnormal thermal effects (heat, cold)
- Electricity
- Suffocate
- Strangulation
- Poison

There is probably no form of violent impact that per se speaks for a certain type of origin, and the differentiation between self-

S. Ahne et al., *Forensic aspects in emergency medicine*,
https://doi.org/10.1007/978-3-662-65949-6_5

infliction, third-party infliction and accident is always a particular challenge in forensic medical assessment. Sometimes the question must remain open.

Indications of an origin by own hand are:

- Grouped injuries
- No defensive injuries
- Quiet injury pattern

Speak for a creation by foreign hand:

- Irregular anatomical distribution of injuries
- Injuries of the vertex region (above the “hat brim line”)
- Injuries to central parts of the face and ears
- Injuries to the ulna-side of the forearms (“defence injury”)
- Several different types of mechanical force

An anatomical distribution typical for the respective assumed cause of the accident and occasionally rather extensive injuries are indicative of an accidental origin. Typical for falls are injuries over protruding bony parts, such as the knees, elbows, shoulders, hips or chin, occiput or lateral parts of the forehead.

In the forensic context, vitality (from vitalitas [Latin] = life force) means that a finding was made while the victim was alive, i.e. with preserved circulation, respiration and metabolism. Some findings (such as bloody footprints or drip marks in the case of cuts) prove a preserved capacity for action, and occasionally actions borne by consciousness can be reconstructed through the traces at the crime scene. However, differentiation from agonal, supravital or postmortem emergence can be difficult, particularly as the transitions are fluid. Autoptic vital signs are haemorrhages or embolisms indicating preserved circulation, deep aspirations, especially in combination with acute emphysema as a sign of preserved respiratory activity, the swallowing of foreign bodies and their intestinal onward transport, and tissue reactions (swelling, inflammation, thrombosis, wound healing).

5.2 Blunt Force

Case Histories

In the night from Saturday to Sunday, the emergency services were called out in front of a large discotheque, where several drunken young men got into a physical altercation. Only with great effort and the use of pepper spray did the police manage to separate the opponents. As an ambulance crewyou take one patient into your vehicle, as according to passers-by he had taken most of the punches and kicks, while a second vehicle crew looks after the other participants. Your patient is permanently squinting his eyes due to irritation from the pepper spray. The whole face seems swollen, the bleeding from the burst lower lip has already stopped. On repeated questioning, the patient states pain in the region of the ribs and in the abdomen; according to him, the head would "burst" in a moment. The patient, who appears very upset and agitated, is rather averse to a more detailed examination, "he would have had enough trouble tonight". You attribute the affective derailment to the patient's generous consumption of alcohol. Since the vital signs are stable, you decide to transport the patient without an emergency doctor on scene to the nearest appropriate hospital with the working hypothesis of "suspected cranial and thoracic contusion and exclusion of abdominal trauma with concomitant alcohol intoxication." One hour after this mission, you are called as an emergency ambulance to the surgical outpatient department of the target hospital, because your former patient has been diagnosed with a severe epidural hemorrhage and is now also so vigilance-diminished that he had to be intubated by the emergency team called in – your mission is the emergency transfer to the already pre-informed neurosurgery of the responsible university hospital.

You have a bad feeling because the doctor on duty draws your attention to the large haematoma on the skullcap above the brim of the hat, which you did not describe before, as well as the present pupillary deviation. The patient always squinted his eyes, but now it is difficult for you to convince him that the pupil difference must have developed in the course of the operation.

5.2.1 Introduction

Blunt force is defined as *an impact of a blunt-edged surface against the human body.* We are all familiar with minor blunt force injuries from everyday life, such as hitting a table or tripping and falling to one's knees. However, they can also be severe and life-threatening, such as from a blow to the head with a hammer (Fig. 5.1) or from a fall from a great height onto a hard floor.

5.2.2 External Injuries

Blunt force injuries to the skin are caused by compressive or tensile stress (Graph 5.1).

The resulting injuries are skin reddening, skin bleeding, skin subcutaneous bleeding, abrasions, contusion wounds, lacerations or contusion lacerations. It should be noted, however, that the

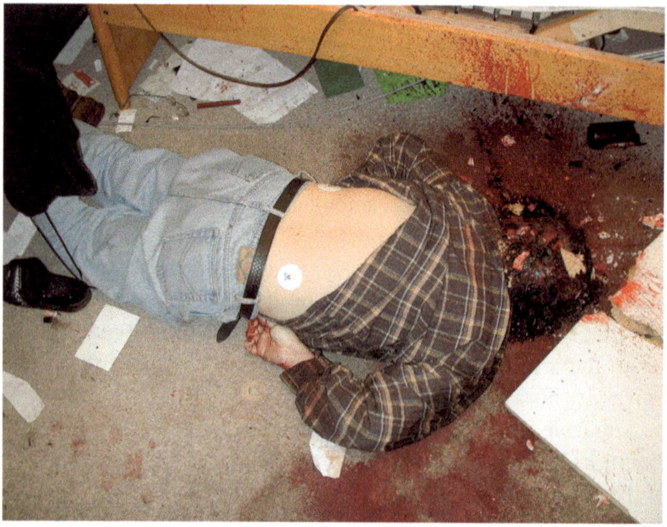

Fig. 5.1 Homicide by multiple blunt force trauma to the head. The bloodstain distribution pattern suggests that at least some blows against the head occurred at the site where the victim was found

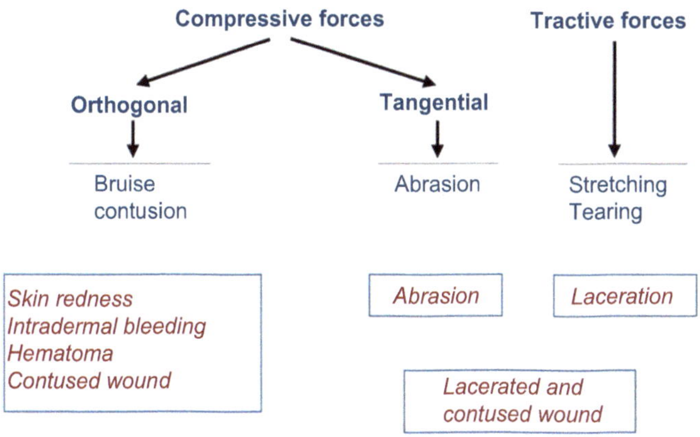

Graph 5.1 Comparisson of compressive and tractive forces

absence of externally visible injuries does not exclude internal injuries, even of a more serious nature. This applies particularly to children.

5.2.2.1 Reddening of the Skin

Reddening of the skin is caused by an increase in the amount of blood in the vessels of the skin after comparatively minor blunt force. They are often visible for only a short time (minutes to hours), during which they gradually fade. They may be shaped to reflect the imprint of the impacting object, both as a positive imprint and as a negative imprint.

5.2.2.2 Intradermal Bruises

Intradermal bruises are caused by ruptures of vessels in the dermis, usually due to a sudden increase in blood volume when the skin is pressed into the indentation of objects. These can be soft objects, such as the clothing worn (Fig. 5.2), but also firm profiles such as shoe soles or depressions in car tyres. The hemorrhages are usually punctate, bright red, sharply demarcated, and rarely are extensive. Occasionally, the punctate hemorrhages may be so close together as to give an areal impression. They are usually less impressive than the larger and more intensely colored skin

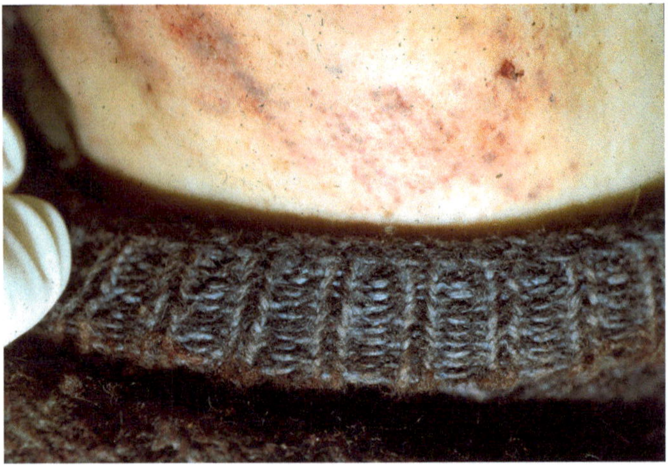

Fig. 5.2 Intracutaneous bleeding in the form of a clothing imprint mark. Negative imprint of the turtleneck sweater after kicks to the neck

subcutaneous bruises, but they indicate the site of a violent impact. They are often configured in a pattern-like fashion, representing the negative imprint of the causative object (Fig. 5.3). A particular form is double-striped, parallel, red skin discolorations caused by blows with a narrow, elongated object. These cause the vessels in the skin to be compressed under the percussion tool and blood to be displaced to the edges of the compressed skin area on both sides. The double contour imprint of the impactor may be visible for a short time as reddening of the skin (Sect. 5.2.2.1) or, in the case of rupture of the intradermal vessels as a result of volume overload, as intradermal bruises for up to a few days.

5.2.2.3 Bruises

Skin subcutaneous hemorrhages, also called hematomas, suffusions or sugillations or simple bruises, are localized in the subcutaneous fat tissue. They can occur at the site of the primary force or away from it. An example of a hemorrhage away from the primary force is the bilateral black eye following a fall on the back of the head. In this case, pressure displacements inside the skull

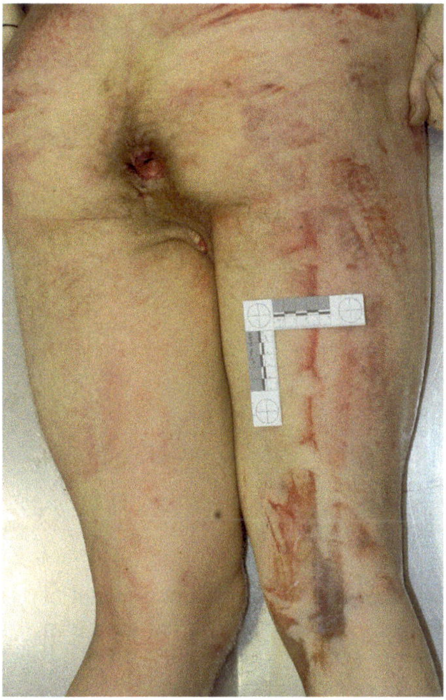

Fig. 5.3 Tyre imprint after being rolled over by a truck

can lead to fractures of the orbital roofs with subsequent bleeding into the retroorbital tissue. These hemorrhages are then also visible externally (Fig. 5.4). At the site of the violent impact, haematomas are caused by vascular ruptures in the subcutaneous fatty tissue, usually in the context of bruising. Since the subcutaneous fatty tissue is built as a loose lobular structure, the hemorrhages can spread over a large area and also migrate over time. For example, bruises originally localized in the jaw area may slip toward the neck as a result of gravity. Hematomas are resorbed over time, which is associated with a change in color. The fresh hematoma is generally blue-purple in color (depending on the thickness of the hemorrhage and the skin hue) and changes to green and then yellow color over time. Since hematomas are degraded from their

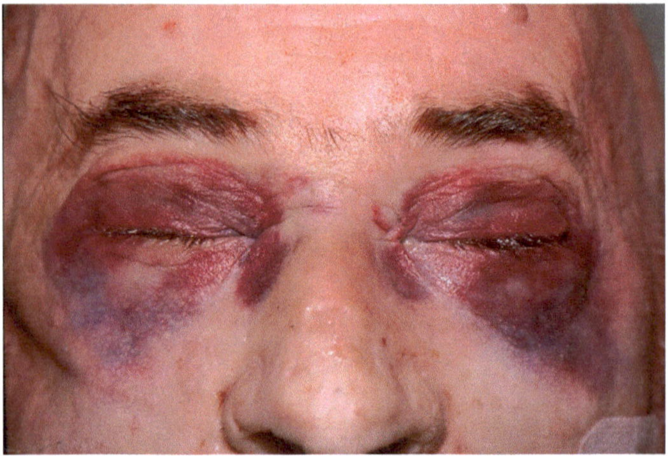

Fig. 5.4 bilateral black eyes: Underbleeding of the lid membranes on both sides

edges, this is also where the color change first becomes visible, combined with an increasing blurring of the edges.

5.2.2.4 Abrasions

Abrasions are caused by the tangential application of force. Depending on the strength and angle of the applied force, layers of skin are pushed away in the direction of the applied force. The end of the abrasion is characterised by an abrasion moraine, to which wallpaper-like, pushed-together skin rolls are attached which is also called the terminal epidermal tag. In the case of a fresh injury, wound secretion emerges, which can also be bloody in the case of a deeper abrasion, since the skin capillaries there are damaged if the dermis is involved. Over time, a yellow-brownish scab develops from the wound secretion, which dries up and covers the wound on the outside. The duration of wound healing depends on the area and depth of the abrasion. The following Table 5.1 gives a rough indication of the time required.

In cases of death, fresh abrasions dry up, as no wound healing takes place post mortem, and take on a honey-yellow (in skin areas with little blood) to reddish-brown colour (in skin areas with

Table 5.1 Time trends

Findings	Time
Bleeding time	Few minutes
Soft scab	1 h
Solidified scab	1 day
Fall of the scab	7–10 days

a lot of blood) and a firm, leathery consistency. Such desiccations are not a vital sign, as postmortem epidermal loss also leads to corresponding findings. Postmortem desiccations have the same morphology as in the case of non-survived abrasion during life.

5.2.2.5 Contused Wounds

Contused wounds are caused by compressive forces that are so strong that the continuity of the skin is severed. Contused wounds occur mainly in areas of the body where bony structures tend to be superficial, so that the skin and underlying soft tissue layers are contused between the blunt-edged object and the bone. They are localized at the site of primary force and are characterized by irregular wound edges with a fringe of abrasion or desiccation and bridges of tissue at the depth of the wound. The wound edges may be underminable.

5.2.2.6 Lacerations

Lacerations occur away from the site of primary force due to overstretching of the skin. They are characterised by smooth, non-abrasive wound edges and tissue bridges in depth. The course of the wound edge is often irregular in itself, somewhat wavy and not as straight as in a cut wound. Often several tears are found next to each other, especially when only the outer layers of the skin are affected. Such injuries are found, for example, in the groin of pedestrians who have been hit from behind (Fig. 5.5).

5.2.2.7 Contused and Lacerated Wounds

Contused laerations are a combination of contused wounds and lacerations and are located at the site of the primary force. They

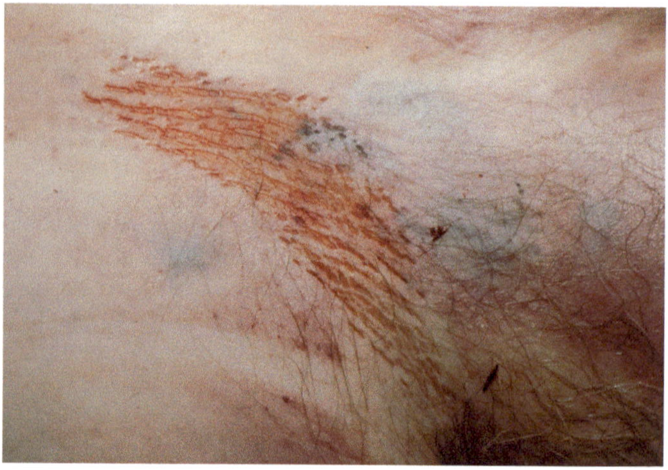

Fig. 5.5 Overstretching lacerations of the skin in the right groin region of a pedestrian as a result of a powerful car impact on the legs from behind

occur almost exclusively on the scalp, as the skin there is firmly fused with the underlying tendon plate (galea aponeurtica), which means that the scalp is not very mobile. Compressive forces, such as from a blow, bruise the tissue, while marginal tensile forces act on the tissue in the immediate vicinity until it tears to relieve the pressure. The contused parts of the wound lie centrally and are characterised by scraped wound edges (Fig. 5.6). The same morphological criteria apply to these as to the lacerations. In terms of size and shape, the scraped portions reflect the contact surface of the impinging tool: In the case of force acting over a wide area (e.g. a fall with the head striking the ground), the wounds tend to be roundish-oval and show broad scraping edges and often several marginal cracks that may extend in different directions. Narrow, angular structures (such as the edge of a table) are more likely to

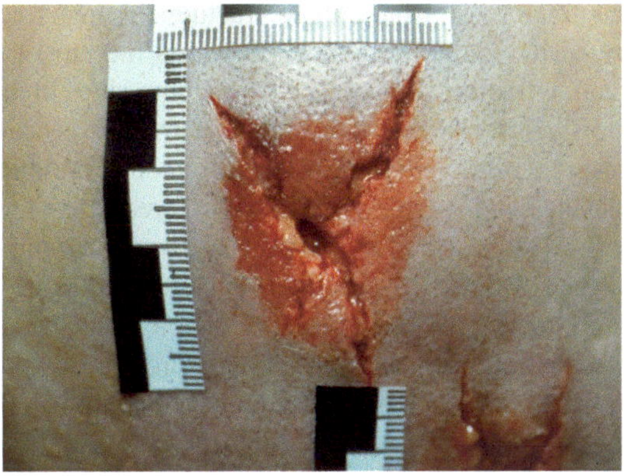

Fig. 5.6 Multiple lacerated and contused wound of the scalp after impact with a bottle

result in straight, narrow skin tears with millimetre-wide abrasion fringes and rather short tears originating from the wound angles.

5.2.3 Internal Injuries

5.2.3.1 Cranium

Fractures of the skull occur due to local or global deformation. Accordingly, a distinction is made between bending fractures (local deformation of the skull) and burst fractures (global deformation of the skull). **Burst fractures** are mainly localized in the base of the skull and may involve the lateral portions of the calvaria. They are the typical consequences of falls with impact of the skull on the ground. The course of the fracture line indicates the vector of the force impact: A compression in the longitudinal direction leads to a longitudinal fracture, a compression in the transverse direction leads to a transverse fracture. A special form is the annular fracture around the foramen magnum, which can occur, for example, in traffic accidents with frontal collision, if the torso is fixed in the seat by the belt during sudden deceleration, but the head continues to move forward due to inertia. There are several forms of **bending fractures**: simple fracture, globe fracture, pond fracture and buttonhole fracture. Simple fracture is characterized by simple fracture lines and is the most common form of calotte fracture. It is caused by circumscribed blunt force. The globe fracture is characterized by a fracture system with radial and circular fracture lines, which is remotely reminiscent of the meridians of a globe. It is the result of a force acting on a large area. The pond fracture and the buttonhole fracture are impression fractures, in which the edges of the fracture are stepped (pond fracture) or punched out like holes (buttonhole fracture).

Injuries to the brain caused by blunt force are divided into translation trauma and rotation trauma. In the case of **translational trauma,** the force is transmitted in a straight line in the head and is reflected radiologically and morphologically in so-called cortical contusions, which are accompanied by subarachnoid and subdural haemorrhages (see below). The contusions occur on the side facing the impact (coup) and on the opposite impact side (contrecoup). Latter is typically at the base of the brain, very often at the temporal and frontal lobes. **Rotational trauma** results from a rapid rotational movement of the head in the horizontal axis. This results in the occurrence of shear forces, which can lead to the rupture of bridging veins on the one hand, and to diffuse axonal damage in the medullary layer of the brain on the other.

Craniocerebral trauma is classically divided into different forms according to its severity and the morphological or radiological findings: The lightest is the head contusion **(contusio capitis)**, a trivial trauma against the head, in which there may be blood underflow or even sometimes violently bleeding crush lacerations. Since the scalp is well innervated, the injury is also usually quite painful. However, it is important that consciousness is not affected. The next stage is the mildest form of brain injury, the concussion (**commotio cerebri**). It is a central nervous functional disorder that is not morphologically or radiologically associated with tangible focal injuries. Signs of commotio cerebri are a brief disturbance of consciousness with retrograde amnesia, which is not always remembered by the victim. This is followed by nausea, vomiting and headache. Brain contusion **(contusio cerebri)** results in demonstrable damage to the brain, such as cortical hemorrhages and subarachnoid hemorrhages. Clinically, patients are conspicuous by prolonged unconsciousness. The damage heals with defect formation. The cerebral contusion **(Compressio cerebri)** is the result of an increase in pressure in the brain due to space-occupying haemorrhages or severe (malignant) oedema. Radiologically as well as macromorphologically, it is characterized by brain swelling with elapsing of the surface and flattening of the convolutions. In unilateral processes there is displacement of the midline. Since the brain can only expand upwards and laterally to a limited extent due to the limitation by the calvaria, the brain stem is displaced towards the foramen magnum in the course of the disease, which leads to entrapment of the medulla oblongata with the respiratory centre and to central regulatory failure.

Clinically, the different degrees of traumatic brain injury (TBI) are determined using the Glasgow Coma Scale (GCS) and differentiated into mild, moderate and severe TBI.

Intracranial hemorrhages are classified according to their location:

Epidural hemorrhages almost always result from a skull fracture of the temporal region with tearing of the meningeal artery. On CT, they present as lenticular hemorrhages that compress the brain in the neighborhood. In more severe hemorrhages, midline displacement occurs. Typical of epidural hemorrhage is the so-called free interval between the trauma with brief unconsciousness and the onset of intracranial pressure symptoms (neurological deficits, dilatation of the ipsilateral pupil). The lethality is 5–10% (Graph 5.2b).

Subdural hemorrhages lie beneath the hard meninges and occur in isolation in rotational traumas of the head with injuries to the bridging veins between the surface of the brain and the sickle-shaped blood vessel, as concomitant hemorrhages in skull fractures, or combined with subarachnoid hemorrhages in contusions of the cerebral cortex. A typical example of the occurrence of isolated subdural haemorrhages is the shaking trauma of an infant, in which there is tearing of the bridging veins as a result of violent swaying of the head back and forth (Graph 5.2c).

Traumatic **subarachnoid haemorrhages** (SAB) are – in contrast to spontaneous SAB, which originate from ruptures of the

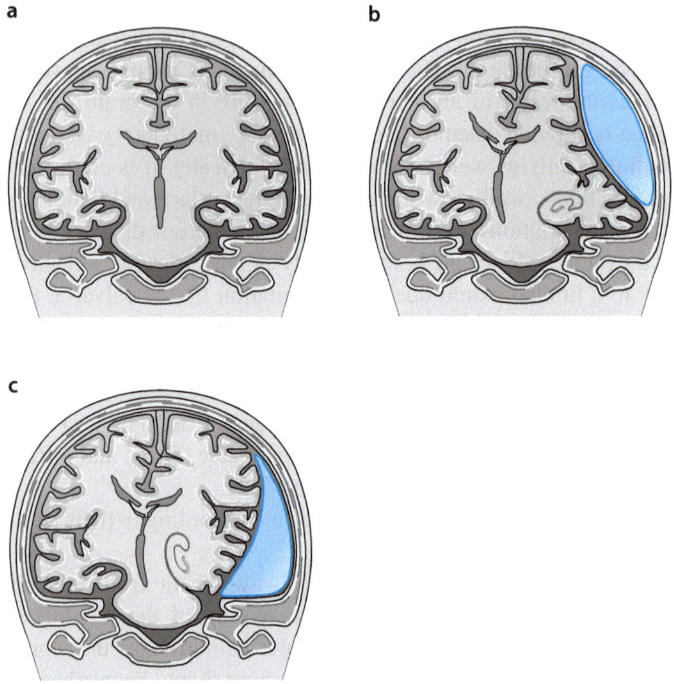

Graph 5.2 Location of epi- and subdural hemorrhages

cerebral basal arteries – consequences of cerebral contusions. As the arachnoid often ruptures, they are usually combined with subdural haemorrhages.

Intracerebral hemorrhages without connection to the brain surface are extremely rare as a result of trauma. They occur only with massive rotational accelerations of the head. In the reconstruction of an accident they raise many questions, because it is difficult to clarify whether the patient got the intracerebral haemorrhage due to the accident or whether a mass haemorrhage in the sense of a haemorrhagic insult was the trigger for the accident.

A common type of injury is a fall on the back of the head. In this case there is a classic constellation of findings:

- Bruising of the occiput of the head
- Simple skull fracture with fracture centre at the back of the head and continuation into the skull base
- Longitudinal skull base fracture
- Cerebral cortex contusion foci (contrecoup) at the base of frontal brain and possibly temporal lobe
- Concomitant subdural and subarachnoid hemorrhage at the base of the brain
- Fractures of the orbital roofs
- Bilateral black eyes

5.2.3.2 Face and Neck

Injuries typical of blunt force trauma to the face include periorbital heamatoma, contusion wounds or contusion lacerations in the eyebrow region, abrasions and/or heamatomas of the cheeks and zygomatic arch region or the jaw angles. Fractures of the zygomatic bones, nasal bone, or mandible may result from fisticuffs to the face. According to *LeFort,* fractures of the facial skull are divided into grades I–III, although this classification only tells us something about the origin of the fracture to a limited extent (Graph 5.3). A special form is the blow-out fracture, in which blunt force against the eye causes a fracture of the orbita.

In cases of blunt force trauma to the neck, fractures of the larynx and contusions of the thyroid gland occur most frequently in addition to external injuries such as hematomas or abrasions. Less common are injuries to the internal carotid artery (usually incomplete rupture or wall dissection). Complete rupture is likely to occur only with massive force and is immediately fatal, whereas incomplete rupture has a highly variable appearance and is therefore easily overlooked. Injuries to the larynx pose a risk of airway obstruction with subsequent suffocation because of edema formation and bleeding.

5.2.3.3 Trunk and Extremities

Spine It takes relatively strong force to injure the spine, unless there are pre-existing conditions such as osteoporosis. The danger

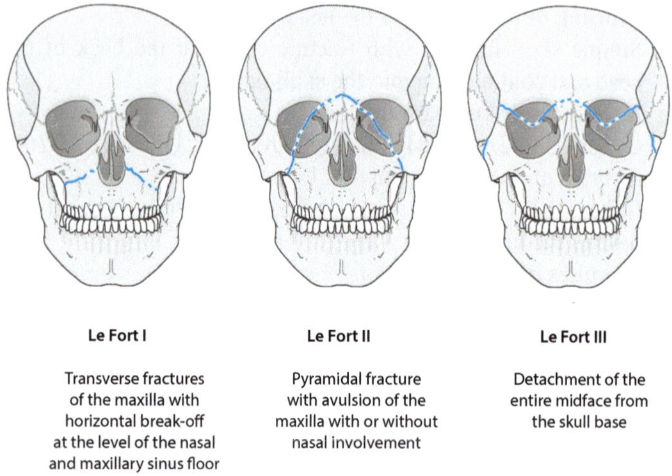

Graph 5.3 Le Fort fractures Typ 1-3

is a contusion to the point of entrapment and/or an avulsion of the spinal cord. Depending on the level, paralysis up to tetraplegia may result. The so-called "neck fracture" is caused by a fracture of the cervical vertebrae C1/2 or a luxation of the head. In this case, the brain stem and cervical medulla are damaged to such an extent that death occurs quickly. However, this is a rare event.

Thorax The internal organs of the thorax are protected by the ribcage, but not from more forceful impact. Circumscribed, but also extensive force can lead to rib fractures. We speak of serial rib fractures when several adjacent ribs are fractured, and of partial rib fractures when one or more ribs are broken several times. In children, bruising of the heart and lungs can occur due to the particularly elastic connections of the ribs without fractures. Cardiac ruptures occur with massive blunt force trauma to the precordial region. A typical example is a traffic accident in which the driver is not wearing a seat belt and the upper body hits the steering wheel. Rupture of the aorta is more common than cardiac rupture. This is a typical deceleration trauma from higher speed. An example of this is a fall from a great height. The site of rupture is at the level of the aortic isthmus. The lung can either be bruised or crushed or, in the case of rib fractures, can also be impaled by free fracture ends. This may result in a haematothorax, a pneumothorax or a haematopneumothorax.

Abdomen In contrast to the thorax, the organs of the abdomen are not protected from the front by bony structures. Nevertheless, especially the organs of the mid-abdomen are rarely injured by blunt force trauma. The liver and the spleen rupture particularly frequently. Rupture of the urinary bladder is rather rare, unless it is full to bursting at the moment of force, or bruising/rupture of the pancreas. When force is applied from behind, such as by kicking, the kidneys are often affected. In general, injuries to organs with capsules, such as the spleen, must be considered for the risk of two-stage rupture and such patients must be monitored closely. Ruptures of hollow organs, such as the stomach or intestines, are rare and are most likely to occur when the abdomen is kicked or (for example, in cases of child abuse) the trunk is severely crushed. Not so rare, especially in traffic accidents, are bleeding and tearing of the mesentery. Very rarely, blunt force against the abdomen can lead to a rupture of the aorta, but in this case there is often previous damage to the aorta. In pregnant women, damage to the fetus or rupture of the uterus and detachment of the placenta may occur.

Pelvis **Pelvic** fractures most commonly occur in traffic accidents or falls from a height. Pelvic fractures are divided into type A, B and C. Type A are stable breaks or cracks at the edge of the pelvis. Type B fractures are also known as “open book” fractures because there is a break in the symphysis or anterior pelvic ring and the pelvis can be “opened up” on clinical examination. Type C fractures are vertically unstable in addition to rotational instability. The problem with unstable pelvic fractures (type B and C) is usually severe bleeding from the vessels supplying the pelvis. They cannot be squeezed off, as is the case with the femoral artery, so that preclinical pressure from outside against the pelvis is the only way to minimize this bleeding.

Extremities The long tubular bones break due to bending, twisting or compression. The older the patient, the more easily bones break. A typical extremity injury in the elderly is the femoral neck fracture after a fall. A typical type of fracture in pedestrian accidents is the Messerer wedge fracture of the tibia at the point where the impact was made by the bumper of the vehicle involved in the accident. In this case, the base of the wedge is on the side where the impact occurred, with the arrow pointing in the same direction as the acting force vector.

5.3 Sharp Force

Case Histories

At around 2 a.m. you are alerted to a reported robbery of a taxi. You are already expected by the police officers who have arrived before you, so that you do not have to take any further measures of self-protection. You find the 46-year-old taxi driver covered in blood and in haemorrhagic shock, so that you and your team decide to transfer the patient to the ambulance as a crash rescue. While venous access and infusion solutions are being prepared in the ambulance, you cut open the clothing of the conditionally responsive man. You notice several small cuts on both hands. In addition, you discover a heavily bleeding gaping wound on the right side of the neck, a cut on the right upper arm and a stab wound on the right side of the thorax. Since on auscultation the respiratory sound on the right side is weakened and breathing is restricted, you decide, after wound care including manual compression of the neck wound and creation of two large-volume venous accesses, to create a Bülau thoracic drainage in the 4th ICR on the right side under analgesia. Approximately one liter of blood is drained from the drainage. Due to your measures, the respiratory situation improves considerably under oxygen insufflation and after 1.5 litres of crystalloid and colloid infusion solutions, the blood pressure rises to 90 mm Hg systolic, so that you can start the emergency transport to the shock room of a hospital with ENT department and thoracic surgery. Before this, you are asked by the police officers, who are under great pressure to find the perpetrator, what you can say about the injuries and the presumed course of events, as the patient is not fit to be questioned. You state that there are several potentially life-threatening cuts and stab wounds. In addition, you suggest that because the injuries are strictly to the right and there are defensive injuries to both sides of the hand, it could be that the attack occurred in the taxi and that the driver probably fought back.

Two days later you learn that the patient has confirmed your suspicions during an interrogation in the intensive care unit. The perpetrator had asked the driver to stop and hand over the cash box. Despite the threatening situation, the driver tried to snatch the knife held out to threaten the attacker, whereupon the perpetrator abruptly struck his victim with the knife.

5.3.1 Introduction

Sharp force refers to the impact of objects that either have a sharp, cutting edge or are pointed. Accidental injuries from sharp force are very common and familiar to all of us from everyday life, although these injuries are usually superficial and do not require treatment. More serious injuries are less common. Here, accidents no longer dominate, but intentionally inflicted injuries must be considered; so-called stabbings are not uncommon in emergency services. But self-injurious or suicidal acts caused by sharp violence are not rarities either. Deaths from sharp violence are comparatively rare. Among these, homicides dominate, being about five times more common than completed suicides. Fatal accidents due to sharp violence are rarities. The main instruments used in serious injuries are knives and broken glass. Less frequently, objects such as scissors, pens, ice picks, screwdrivers or similar are used.

5.3.2 Wound Morphology

In the case of injuries caused by sharp force, a distinction is made between a stab, a cut and a sharp blow.

A **stitch** is caused by a pointed instrument that is guided orthogonally to the surface of the body. The wound channel is deeper than the wound gap is long.

An **incision** is made by a cutting tool that is guided tangentially to the surface of the body. The wound is longer than deep.

A **blow** is caused by a heavy instrument with a cutting edge. The wound can be both long and deep.

All wounds due to sharp violence are characterized by the following morphological details:

- Smooth, often straight, adaptable wound edges
- No scrape hem
- No tissue bridges in the depth of the wound

Most stab wounds are elliptical or almond-shaped (Fig. 5.7). Depending on where the stab wound is located, the wound edges diverge to varying degrees. This has to do with the skin tension lines (Relaxed skin tension lines, RSTL). Normally, there are no abrasions or contusions around the stab wound. An exception to this is a bruise line, which can occur due to a puncture to the hilt of the weapon and can be indicative of a homicide. Most crime tools are single-edged, resulting in different shapes of wound angles. The wound angle pointing to the cutting side is pointed, in the case of a double-edged tool, two pointed wound angles are found accordingly. The back of the instrument also leaves a characteristic wound angle, which can be rounded, angular or V-shaped. The V-shaped angle is clearly created when the edges of the back are particularly sharp. If the weapon is not pulled out completely vertically, a carver-like protrusion of the wound angle occurs on the cutting side. Axial rotation of the weapon in the wound produces V and L configurations (Graph 5.4). The V-shaped configuration is also known as the “fishtail”. The main danger in stab wounds is acute volume deficiency shock due to external or internal bleeding. Stabbings to the chest also pose the risk of pericardial tamponade or hemato- or pneumothorax. In stabs to the neck, in addition to blood loss from injury to the arterial or venous vessels, there may be blood aspiration from injury

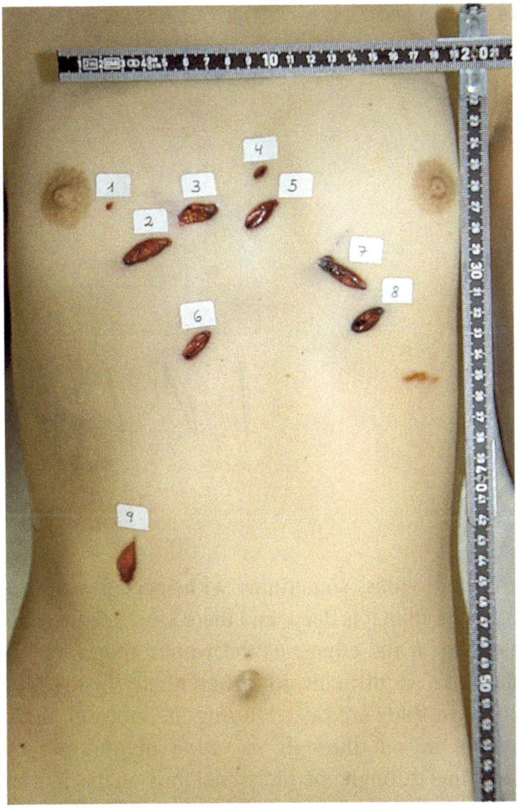

Fig. 5.7 Homicide by numerous knife wounds in the chest and abdomen

to the trachea and air embolism from opening of the jugular veins. For the development of an air embolism, as little as 70–150 ml of air is sufficient. The penetration of air can be heard auscultatorily as a kind of mill noise if it is suspected. The victim himself hears a bubbling sound. Rather rarely, there is a stabbing into the neck with injury of the cervical medulla or into the skull with possible intracranial bleeding.

The wound edges of incised wounds also gape to different degrees, depending on how deep they are and how they run in relation to the skin tension lines. The angles of the wound are

Graph 5.4 Stab wound configurations

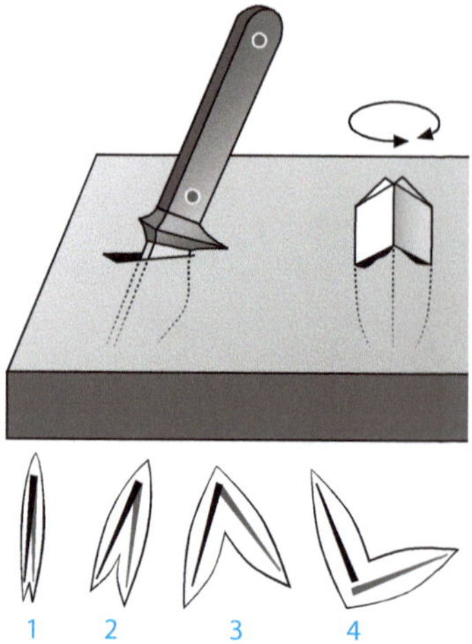

pointed on both sides, sometimes with incised extensions. The wound is longer than it is deep, and there are often no accompanying hematomas at the edges, as the wound may bleed outward. This can make it difficult to differentiate from postmortem wounds. If skin folds are raised during the incision, the fold valleys may not be cut through, resulting in multiple incisional wounds in a line through one incisional movement. In most cases, incisional wounds are not fatal because they rarely injure the larger, deeper vessels. They are particularly significant in suicides. Typical sites are the wrists, the crook of the elbow and the neck (Fig. 5.8).

Puncture wounds or cuts made of glass are a special case, as glass fragments are very thick compared to a knife and often have not one but two cutting edges on the fracture surface, namely a slightly protruding edge on each edge of the cullet. This results in superficial cuts or wound angle extractors often consisting of two parallel scores. Furthermore, the wound edges are occasionally serrated.

A cutting tool has a cutting side and a high dead weight. Typical representatives are axes, hatchets or machetes. Wounds

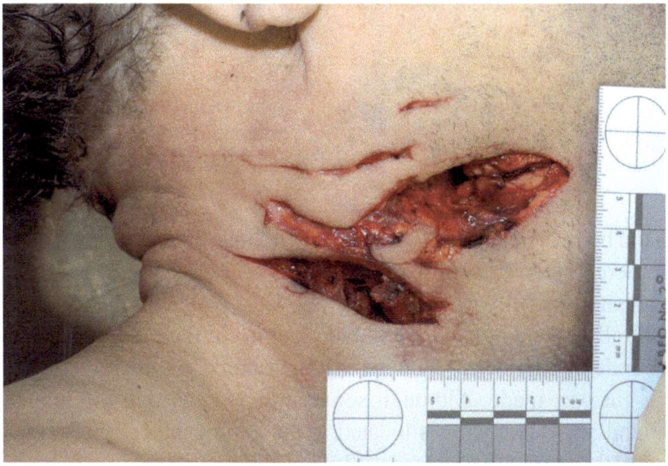

Fig. 5.8 Suicide by stabbing and cutting of the neck. Typical are the accompanying, rather superficial cuts and the parallel alignment

caused by a blow are usually straight, the edges of the wound may be bruised or scraped, and bones may suffer nick-like injuries and impression fractures, especially of the skull, against which the blows are usually struck. Causes of death are also here mainly the internal and external bleeding, possibly also open craniocerebral trauma.

5.3.3 Criminal Aspects

It is only possible to a very limited extent to deduce the murder weapon from the wound dimensions. Stab wounds can be larger, the same size or smaller than the blade width of the murder weapon. The puncture canal can also be longer than the actual blade length due to compression of the soft tissues. Also, the depth of penetration can only be used to a limited extent to infer the force with which the stab was made. The main resistance to a stabbing tool is offered by the skin and the clothing worn over it. Once these have been overcome, the resistance of the soft tissues

Table 5.2 Differences between self-provision and third-party provision

Self-provided	Third-party accommodation
Grouped injuries	Distributed injuries
Typical: Heart region (Fig. 5.9), neck, wrist flexor sides	Typical: Back, skull, lower extremities
Trial injuries	Defensive injuries

in the body is negligible. However, it will take a great deal of force to pierce bony structures such as the sternum or calvaria. If the blade has not fully penetrated the body, the puncture channel will naturally be shorter than the blade length. In the case of incised wounds, it cannot be deduced with certainty in which direction the cut was made. Although some authors state that the longer wound angle extractor is located at the end of the cutting movement, there are also contrary opinions and reports.

It can be difficult to distinguish between self-inflicted suicide and homicide. Criteria for differentiation are listed below (see Table 5.2).

Trial or hesitation injuries are superficial, parallel cuts, usually on the flexor sides of the wrists ("pulse vein cuts"), less frequently in the crooks of the elbows, or on the neck, often in the immediate vicinity of deeper cuts (Figs. 5.10 and 5.11). Alternatively, they may be superficial, punctate stitches in the vicinity of deeper stitches, usually in the cardiac region or on the abdomen. The occurrence of hesitation stitches next to deeper cuts or vice versa is rare and should raise doubts about self-infliction.

Defensive wounds are localized to the hands and forearms. Active defensive wounds are wounds on the palms, the flexor sides of the fingers or in the spaces between the fingers (Fig. 5.12). They occur when the victim attempts to reach for the knife-wielding hand of the attacker in order to wrest the knife away from him. Stab/cut injuries in the first intermetacarpal space are particularly typical. Passive defensive or parry injuries are wounds that have occurred because the arms were held protectively in front of the body. They are most commonly found on the ulnar edges of the forearms, the forearm extensor sides and the backs of the hands.

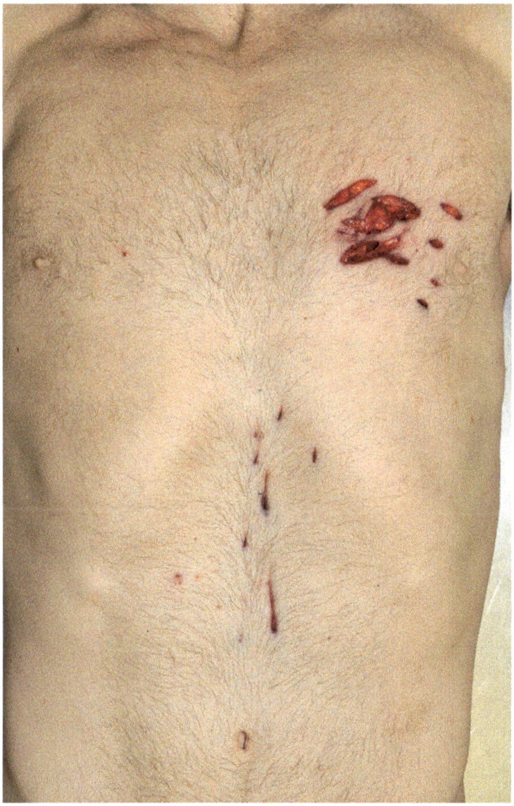

Fig. 5.9 Suicide by stabbing in the cardiac region. The grouped arrangement and the presence of superficial probing or hesitating stabs speak for self-infliction

However, injuries to the palms are not automatically defensive injuries. The attacker can also injure himself if the blade is suddenly braked sharply when stabbing, for example through bone contact, and the knife-wielding hand slips from the handle onto the blade as a result. Depending on the position of the knife, this can result in injuries to the flexor sides of the fingers or the palm of the hand. It is characteristic that, in contrast to defensive injuries, only one (the knife-wielding) hand is injured, that only the

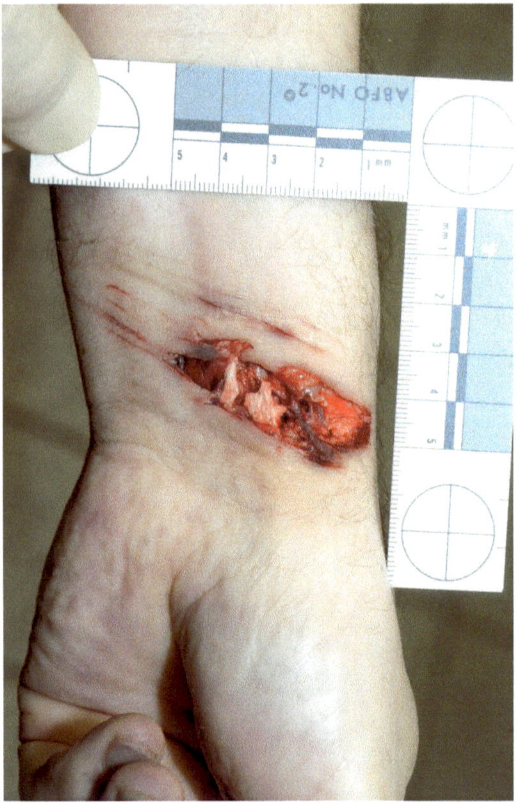

Fig. 5.10 Attempted suicide by pulsar cutting. Characteristic are the superficial trial cuts

palm or the flexor sides of the fingers are affected and that these are transverse to the longitudinal axis of the fingers or to the palm, that the cuts are graduated in a staircase-like manner if several fingers are affected and that the most severe/deepest injury is then on the small-finger side.

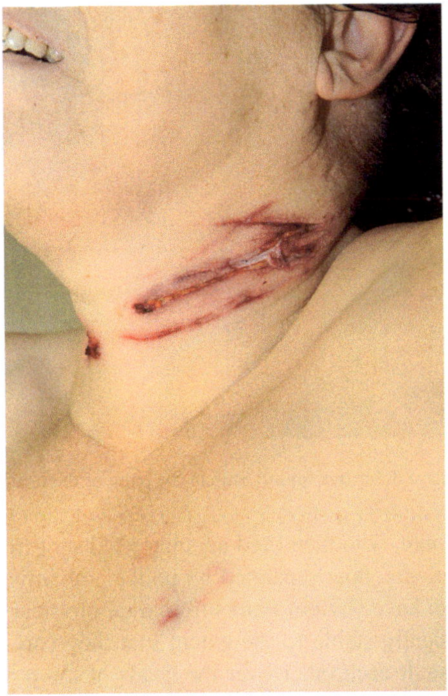

Fig. 5.11 Cut on the neck of a suicidal person. Typical are the multiple, closely juxtaposed, parallel cuts

5.4 Firearms

Case Histories

You are called to a garden settlement as an ambulance with doctor with the mission keyword brawl, probably also use of firearms, police are already on the scene. As always in such operations, you first pay attention to your own safety and, on arrival at the scene, first check with the police whether the scene is safe. Police report that an altercation had occurred between neighbors. Two men went at each other and started fighting. The wife of one of the men became frightened and used a gun to try to get the two to separate. But as the two adversaries continued to fight, one of them bumped

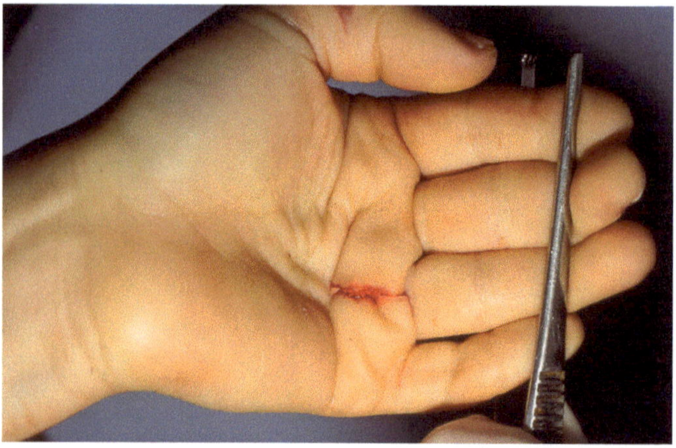

Fig. 5.12 Active defensive injury: Stab in the palm of the hand

into the woman, who then fired an untargeted shot from the gun. The two patients, now separated by police, are sitting outside a gazebo. Both have obvious marks from their physical altercation, but are clinically stable to the extent that they can continue to verbally assault each other over the heads of the police. As the emergency physician, you decide that the Paramedic crew should look at one patient while you examine the other. It soon becomes apparent that your patient has lost two teeth and also may have a fractured nasal bone, but otherwise only abrasions. The paramedic crew's patient has a wrist contusion, abrasions, and an injury to his upper right arm that looks like a bullet hole. You take a closer look at the wound and discover a black discoloration around the wound. As you attempt to place the edges of the wound together, you notice a central loss of substance. The wound is bleeding only moderately, the patient is still very agitated and resists further measures. You decide to transport the patient with your escort to the nearest hospital and order another ambulance for the second patient. During the journey, your patient suddenly complains of increasing shortness of breath and pain in the right side of the chest. You auscultate and note a suspended breath sound on the right side. Upon complete undressing of the upper body, you discover another bullet hole in the thorax below the right axilla and suspect a tension pneumothorax due to the gunshot wound. After you have handed over the patient at the target clinic, however, you ask yourself where the second shot came from, although the police had spoken of only one shot being fired.

5.4.1 Ballistic Principles

Portable firearms are divided into small arms and handguns. Small arms are long-barreled weapons that must be held with two hands, while handguns are short-barreled and can be operated with one hand. **Small arms** are rifles. There is a structural distinction between rifles and shotguns. Rifles have a rifled barrel and are used for single bullets. The rifled barrel, which is made up of raised sections (rifling) and depressions (fields) twisted along the longitudinal axis, gives the bullet a twist that stabilizes it. Shotguns have a smooth bore barrel for firing buckshot. Rifles also include the so-called assault rifles used in the military. **Handguns** include the revolver and the pistol. Revolvers have a rotating drum as a magazine, pistols have a rod magazine usually built into the grip. The firing rate of pistols is higher, because they are so-called self-loaders, in which the case of the fired round is ejected and a new one is inserted into the chamber when the shot is fired.

Rounds are composed of a case and a projectile, the rear part of which is enclosed in the case. The case contains the propellant charge. A primer is installed in the base of the case. When the shot is fired, the firing pin of the weapon hits this plate, causing the propellant charge to ignite and the projectile to accelerate. In buckshot rounds, the projectile consists of numerous small lead pellets separated from the propellant charge by a plug. Single bullets are cylindrically shaped, usually consisting of a lead core partially (partial jacket bullet) or completely (full jacket bullet) enclosed in a metal jacket (usually copper or a copper alloy). However, there are also so-called full jacketed bullets which are not jacketed. These are used, for example, for air guns ("diabolos") or for small-calibre guns. The propellant used today is predominantly cellulose nitrate, which is low in smoke and highly energetic and thus permits higher muzzle velocities. The muzzle velocity for handguns is approximately between 300 and 400 m/s, and between 600 and 1000 m/s for long guns.

5.4.2 Injuries Caused by Projectiles

Projectiles release their kinetic energy into the target and are slowed down in the process. The more energy released, the more severe the wound. Projectiles fired at high muzzle velocity carry more energy, so can produce more severe injuries than projectiles that have been accelerated comparatively fewer. Deformation bullets are designed to deform upon impact with a target – more energy is delivered in this process than by a full metal jacket bullet that is otherwise the same caliber and achieves the same muzzle velocity. The calibre is of secondary importance compared to the muzzle velocity and the deformation capability of the projectile.

When penetrating a body, the projectile is decelerated and releases its energy radially to the firing channel. A temporary wound cavity is created, the diameter of which is many times the diameter of the projectile. As a result, internal injuries also occur away from the actual bullet channel.

Depending on whether and how the projectile hits the body and if necessary penetrates it, a distinction is made between retained missile, shot right through, grazing shot and rebounding shot.

In the case of a **retained missile**, the projectile enters the body, but its energy is no longer sufficient to leave the body again. The projectile remains in the body. It often gets stuck under the skin on the opposite side.

A **shot right through** is when the bullet also leaves the body. There is a bullet exitwound. The shot channel is usually straight. However, the projectile can also be deflected by bone. This is particularly common in the area of the skull. In 10–25% of the cases, so-called angular and ring shots occur. In the case of an angle shot, the projectile hits the bone surface at an angle and is deflected back at an angle. A ring shot occurs on concave bone surfaces, such as in the skull or on the inside of the ribs. The projectile gets a continuous change of direction.

In a **two-segment shot**, the projectile penetrates a body part and then re-enters the body of the same victim, e.g., shot through the upper arm and penetrating the thorax.

A **grazing shot** typically causes channel-shaped injuries. The "shot channel" is completely open.

A **rebounding shot** occurs with dull projectiles that hit the body but do not produce a wound, such as rubber bullets. Nevertheless, internal injuries can occur here.

The distinction between an entrance bullet wound and an exit wound can be made on the basis of typical wound characteristics. An **entrance bullet wound** consists of a tissue defect (i.e. the wound edges are not adaptable) with a contusion hem (formerly called "abrasion hem") in which the epidermis is missing. Depending on the angle at which the projectile impacted the skin, the tissue defect is roundish to oval (Fig. 5.13). In terms of size, it corresponds approximately to the diameter of the projectile. A blackish oily ring, called a wiper ring, can sometimes be found on its inner edge if the projectile has not previously penetrated clothing. The wiper ring is caused by the fact that the projectile is coated with a thin layer of oil (gun oil from cleaning the barrel), to which smudge particles then stick after firing.

A **bullet exit wound** does not necessarily have to be present. However, there are also cases in which only one entrance wound but several exit wounds are found. This regularly leads to confusion during the first examination, but can be explained by a disintegration of the bullet. In contrast to the bullet hole, exit wounds are morphologically quite variable. The rule of thumb that is often read or heard, that ricochet wounds are larger than bullet wounds, is not correct. The shape of the wound depends on how the bullet leaves the body, i.e. in what form, whether orthogonal or transverse, whether it carries bone splinters with it, how much energy it still releases and, finally, whether there is any counterpressure on the skin at the point of impact. All these parameters determine the size of the wound, whether there is a visible tissue defect and whether or not the wound edges show accompanying epidermal lesions (Fig. 5.14).

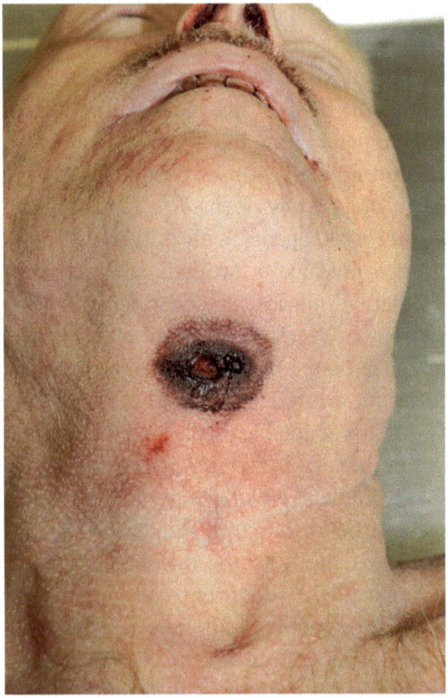

Fig. 5.13 Suicide by gunshot to the bottom of the mouth. Typical features of the entrance bullet wound are the central, round defect, the epidermis-free marginal zone (contusion hem) and the dark-coloured stripping ring or contact ring. Since the weapon was placed directly on the skin when the shot was fired, a muzzle mark has formed

In many thrillers and other films you see that people who are shot immediately become incapacitated, especially if they are shot in the head. However, this does not correspond to reality. If certain brain regions, such as the brain stem, the upper cervical medulla, the cerebellum and other parts of the brain responsible for movement are not primarily destroyed, the victim can still move and is at least capable of short-term actions. This also applies to shots that hit the aorta or the heart, for example. Although death by bleeding to death occurs quickly here, the victim is still capable of acting for the duration of the oxygen reserve

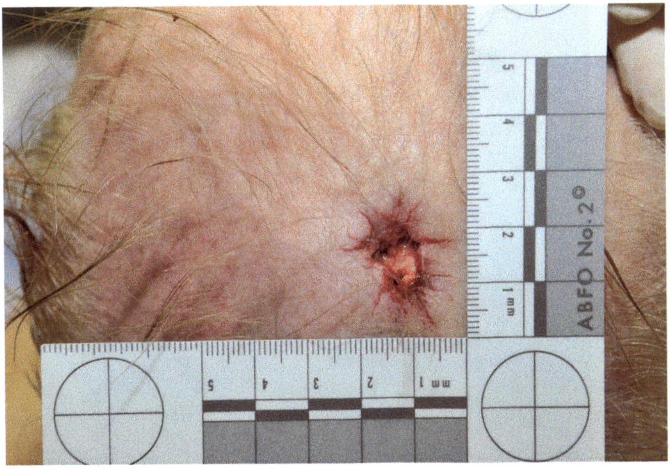

Fig. 5.14 Multi-beam ruptured scab wound in the parietal region (cleaned)

of the brain (about 6–8 s). This explains why some victims are still able to take a few steps despite heart rupture, or why suicides sometimes shoot themselves several times even though the first hit is already fatal.

5.4.3 Criminal Aspects

5.4.3.1 Shot Distance

Depending on the distance of the shot from the point of entry, *a* distinction is made between the *absolute close shot,* the *relative close shot* and the *long shot.*

Absolute Close-Range Shot (contact shot) The muzzle of the weapon is up when the shot is fired, which leads to a change in the bullet morphology. As a result of the muzzle being sealed by the skin, the gunshot gases pass under the skin into the tissue. This is expanded like a balloon by the high pressure and pressed against the barrel muzzle. This causes the weapon's face to be imprinted on the skin, which is known as a *muzzle mark* (Fig. 5.13).

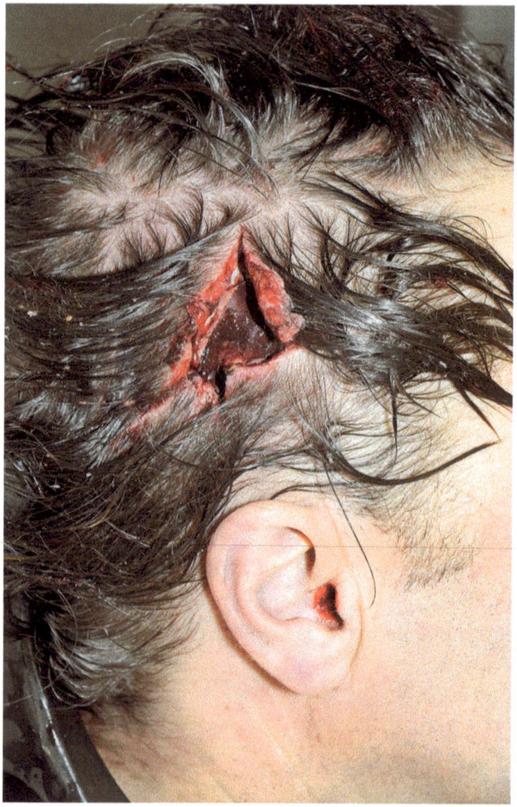

Fig. 5.15 Bullet wound at close range. Due to the high tissue pressure, the skin has been torn open in a star shape and the gunshot residue has been deposited in the initial area of the gunshot channel

Particularly on the head, where the tissue layers above the bone are relatively thin, this causes the skin around the bullet wound to tear open in a star shape (Fig. 5.15). The gunshot residue is deposited in the initial area of the gunshot canal (gunshot cavity).

Relative Close Shot The weapon in this case is not mounted, but a few centimeters to about 1 m away, in any case, at most so far that smoke deposits can be found in the vicinity of the bullet and on the skin. The farther away the shooter is, the larger the soot will be and the lower its intensity will be. The actual distance depends on the smoke characteristics of the weapon and the ammunition. It may have to be determined experimentally.

Long Range Shot A long range shot is when there are no close range signs, i.e., no smoke yard and no powder bursts or buildup.

With shotgun ammunition, the picture changes with increasing distance of the shooter from a central defect to more and more extended sieve-like bullets around the main bullet wound.

5.4.3.2 Shot Placement

In the investigation of gunshot cases, a central question is whether a gunshot wound was self-inflicted, accidental (accidental), or intentionally caused by a third-party perpetrator. This question cannot always be answered conclusively, but the findings on the victim and the circumstances provide clues.

There are typical regions for a suicide. On the head, these include the temple, the forehead, the mouth and the submental area (below the chin). The heart area is also typical for suicidal shooting. Almost always, the barrel is put on during a suicide. In the case of the cardiac region, there is usually no prior disrobing! Examination of the gunshot hand may provide evidence of self-infliction, e.g. blood and tissue particles adhering to the hand (so-called backspatter from the bullet wound). Occasionally, traces of gunshot can be seen with the naked eye. The weapon should be found on site.

Compared to suicidal or homicidal shootings, accidents are relatively rare, but occur again and again. In addition to accidental firing while cleaning a weapon or handling an unsecured firearm as typical accident scenarios, it should also be remembered that occasionally suicides are intended to be dissimulated as accidents, especially in connection with hunting. Typical of accidents in which the shooter himself is hit are relative close-range shots, atypical bullet localizations (compared to a suicide), and longer shot channels in the body to the then fatal organ injuries. The murder weapon is located at the scene.

5.4.3.3 Special Forms

Captive Bolt Gun Bolt guns are used to stun animals for slaughter. The device is designed for multiple use and drives a bolt into the skull with great force and pulls it back again. As a result, no bullet remains in the body. The entry wound is typically punched out, occasionally with two adjoining pockets of gunshot, and the punched out tissue remnant can be found in the depth of the wound. Due to multiple use, the bolt is by no means sanitized, so infection is common if the shot survives.

Explosion Possible injuries from an explosion are divided into four types. *Primary explosion injuries* are caused by the strong overpressure wave and have the effect of barotrauma. Ruptures of the eardrum, ruptures of the lungs with (tension) pneumothorax, ruptures of the liver and spleen, ruptures of the mesentery or intestines, and traumatic amputations of extremities may occur. *Secondary blast injuries* result from flying fragments that act like projectiles. Accordingly, all kinds of bullet-like injuries can occur. The overpressure wave can also cause people to fall and injure themselves or be hit by flying debris. The resulting injuries are called *tertiary blast injuries. Quaternary explosion injuries* are injuries caused by the consequences of the explosion, e.g. fire, radioactive gases or burial under a collapsing building.

Alarm Guns These weapons work with a gas jet, which is fired by igniting firecracker or irritant cartridges. Since April 1, 2003, anyone who wants to carry a scare gun must present a small firearms license. However, the mere possession or purchase of such a weapon is permitted from the age of 18. The gas jet can cause serious injury if fired at an absolute or a relative close range of a few inches. The jet can penetrate the skin and perforate underlying organs. This is particularly dangerous when placed on the skull, because the gas jet is able to penetrate the thin temporal plate and cause damage in the brain tissue.

5.5 Thermal Violence

5.5.1 Heat

Case Histories

It is the middle of the night and you have been standing with an ambulance for hours as a fire watch in front of a burning factory building, because the fire brigade is still in the building with breathing protection. Suddenly and without warning, a respiratory protection team comes out of the building and places a human body in a contorted position in front of your vehicle. Even without an doctor, you can quickly determine death due to the extensive extent and high severity of the burns, including charring. While you are still in the process of notifying a doctor for the official determination of death and the police for the initiation of an investigation into the unnatural manner of death, the first rumours arise at the scene that a violent confrontation must have taken place before death occurred, as the corpse shows large injuries to the abdomen and the "defensive posture" already mentioned. Without participating in the rumors that have arisen, you too are wondering whether there are indications of foul play or whether there is some other explanation for the disfiguring findings.

5.5.1.1 Systemic Heat Damage

The human organism depends on a constant core body temperature of 37 °C on average. Even deviations of a few degrees can have fatal effects, as the metabolism is designed for this narrow temperature range. Heat supply from the outside leads in the long run to an increase of the body core temperature, which the organism tries to compensate mainly by sweating. However, this does not always succeed; in the long run, systemic heat exposure leads to circulatory collapse and functional organ failure. In cases of death due to systemic heat exposure, therefore, no specific findings are found; the diagnosis can only be made by exclusion and in consideration of the circumstances.

Heat Cramps In this case, dehydration and a loss of electrolytes (NaCl) occur during intense physical exertion under great heat (sun, blast furnace, open fire, etc.). The patients complain of cramps in the muscles and have to vomit more often (further loss of fluids!). In the further course, vasodilatation and tachycardia occur. The cramps become life-threatening if the electrolyte shifts in the heart cause disturbances in the conduction of excitation.

Heat Exhaustion/Heat Collapse As with heat cramps, the cause is dehydration. Primary heat collapse results from indirect fluid deprivation during severe vasodilation. Secondary heat collapse results from the loss of fluid due to profuse sweating. Circulatory failure to hypovolemic shock occurs.

Heat Stroke Due to a strong heat supply from the outside and a prevented heat dissipation, the core body temperature rises to over 43 °C. Initially, the red stage occurs, in which the skin is red and dry. If the circulatory system collapses, the grey stage follows with myogenic cardiac insufficiency, twilight states or unconsciousness and seizures.

Sunstroke This is caused by direct sunlight on the head with an increase in temperature on the brain. As the brain reacts very sensitively, the first signs of meningeal irritation and even intracerebral haemorrhage quickly occur.

5.5.1.2 Local Heat Damage

Local heat injuries are burns or scalds. Burns are the consequences of dry heat, such as contact with open flames or hot objects. Scalds result from contact with hot liquids or hot steam. The way heat is transferred to the skin affects the extent of the damage, as do the level of temperature and the duration of exposure. Moist heat conducts much better, so damage to the skin occurs even at lower temperatures. This can be easily understood if one considers that in a Finnish sauna temperatures of 110 °C can be tolerated at very low humidity, whereas in a steam bath temperatures never exceed 45–50 °C. The main difference is the skin's ability to conduct heat. The essential difference is the ability of the skin to keep the effective skin temperature in the tolerable range below 40 °C by evaporation (sweating).

Depending on the depth of the affected skin layers, four different degrees of burns are classified:

Grade 1 – only the epidermis is affected. There is redness, the wound heals without damage.

Grade 2a – here the epidermis is also affected. There is redness and blistering, the wound heals without damage.

Grade 2b – the dermis is also affected. Depending on the depth of damage, there is also reddening or already pallor of the skin and blistering, scars remain. Up to this degree, the wounds are very painful.

Grade 3 – the entire skin is burnt. The wound looks white, leathery, skin appendages such as hair and sweat glands are also affected, due to a destruction of the nerve endings, the patients no longer feel pain, the skin can no longer heal spontaneously.

Grade 4 – Charring; the structures below the skin, such as muscles and bones, are also affected, also no spontaneous healing possible.

Scalds are caused by moist heat in the form of hot liquids or hot steam. They differ from burns by the following points:

- Hairs remain intact. They only burn at temperatures >150 °C
- There is no fourth degree scalding (charring)
- The borders to unaffected skin areas are sharply marked, and the fluid may be seen to run off.
- Clothing may initially protect the skin, but when soaked, clothing increases the duration of exposure to the hot liquid.

To indicate the extent of a burn, the Rule of Nines (Graph 5.5), which involves adding up the area of the burns, has proved useful for many years. This makes it possible to assess whether the

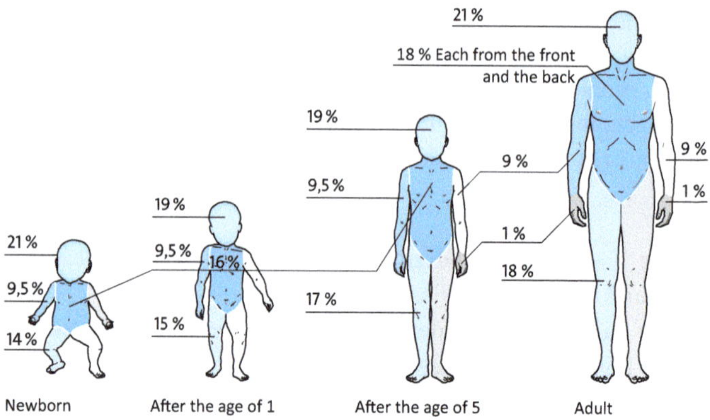

Graph 5.5 Counting burning areas in different ages

patient can be treated in a normal hospital or whether the special treatment of a burn centre is required. To estimate a prognosis of the patient, the burn index is calculated. For this purpose, the age is added with the extent of the 2nd and 3rd degree burns. If this results in a value of <80, there is only a slight danger to life, values between 80 and 120 result in an acute danger to life, and values >120 are rarely survived. As a guide, it can be noted that a value of 100 is survived in 50% with optimal therapy.

5.5.1.3 Fire Deaths

Deaths from fires are either the result of direct exposure to heat through burns to the skin, heat damage to the respiratory tract, and elevation of body temperature or the body's systemic response to it, or the result of inhalation of fire smoke gases, some of which are toxic or corrosive.

In the case of deaths that were recovered after the fire had been extinguished, i.e. that did not die in a hospital as a result of the fire, it must be taken into account that the fire generally lasted beyond death and that the external findings were predominantly post-mortem. This postmortem exposure to fire leads to the destruction of premortem findings and to the appearance of postmortem artifacts due to heat-induced denaturation of proteins, shrinkage of tissues, loss of elasticity, and alteration of the fluid content in tissues. The differentiation of vital findings from postmortem findings is a challenge in forensic medicine.

There are some postmortem changes that occur in burn victims that, if not known, can easily be mistaken for premortem injuries. These changes include:

Skin Splits These splits are usually smooth-edged and can easily be mistaken for cuts. However, they occur postmortem due to shrinkage and loss of elasticity of the skin. In the abdominal area, these tears can lead to the point where the abdominal cavity ruptures.

Pugilistic Attitude Postmortem, the heat causes the muscles and tendons to shrink. This results in the characteristic posture of the corpses, which is reminiscent of a pre-mortem defensive posture (Fig. 5.16). It is characterized by flexion in the elbows and wrists, on the legs by flexion in the knee and hip joints and to a slight external rotation in the hip joints.

Protrusion of the Tongue the tip of the tongue is often protrused between the open rows of teeth and lips, which in combination with the pugilistic attitude reinforces the impression of fight or flight. However, this is also not a vital sign, but an effect of the soft tissue shrinkage of the neck, whereby the tongue is protrused.

The determination of vitality, i.e. exposure to fire during life, and the determination of the cause of death are of central importance in the forensic examination of burnt corpses and are also interlinked. Autoptic signs of vitality are soot ingestion, soot inhalation, increased CO-Hb content in the blood, increased content of cyanides in the blood as well as morphological signs of heat inhalation such as reddening and oedema of the mucous membrane, especially of the larynx.

Not infrequently, the identity of the deceased must also be clarified. The main help here is the dental status. If available, scars from operations and accidents, pathological organ findings or the shape of the frontal sinus can also help. A more complex and costly procedure is the DNA comparison, e.g. with biological relatives.

5.5.2 Cold

Case Histories

You are called to a residential area with the emergency keyword "psychiatric emergency". There you find an elderly man, about

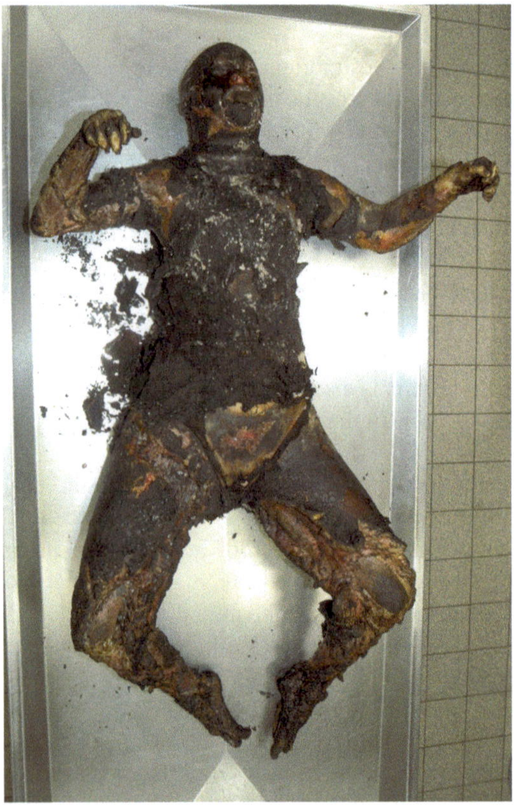

Fig. 5.16 The so-called pugilistic attitude in burnt corpses is the result of postmortem, heat-induced shrinkage of the tendons and musculature

65 years old, standing in the garden of a terraced house, who has undressed down to his underwear and socks despite wintry temperatures of about 5 °C. When you approach him, there is a distinct smell of alcohol. When you ask, the elderly gentleman does not want to put his clothes back on, saying he is warm and everything is fine, he has just had a bit too much to drink. To confirm that everything is all right, he slowly walks away towards the entrance of the house.

What do you do? Do you let him go and just observe whether he actually enters the house? Or do you stop him and insist on an examination in the ambulance, if necessary with the help of the police? Does the emergency call correspond to the situation found?

5.5.2.1 Hypothermia

Hypothermia occurs when the body temperature drops below 36 °C. The body normally tries to prevent cooling by shivering. Normally, the body tries to prevent cooling by shivering. However, this form of heat generation is ineffective because more heat is released at the same time. In newborns and infants, heat is still generated without shivering by burning the so-called brown fatty tissue. Therefore, one should not be lulled into a false sense of security when infants do not shiver. The main way heat is retained is by reducing the blood flow to the skin at the extremities. Thus, only the core of the body is kept at 37 °C. This fact is important for temperature measurement, especially in severely hypothermic persons. Here, only deep rectal or, in the clinic, oesophageal measurements should be taken. Even the tympanal measurement in the ear is no longer accurate enough here; as a self-experiment, a self-measurement after a winter walk is recommended.

When the body temperature drops below 35 °C, it is called cold sickness, which is divided into 4 stages.

Stage 1 – mild hypothermia: core body temperature between 36° and 33 °C, the body's own regulatory measures such as muscle tremors are maximally pronounced but are no longer sufficient. Vital signs include tachycardia and, not infrequently, hyperventilation. The cold-exposed acra are painful.

Neurologically, patients are usually confused and highly agitated. Therefore, this stage is also called the *excitation stage.*

Stage 2 – moderate hypothermia: core body temperature between 33° and 30 °C, "everything slows down": muscle tone decreases, sinus bradycardia now occurs at the heart, central depression increasingly occurs during breathing and pain subsides. Particularly dangerous is the "cold idiocy" that begins here, in which the patients feel a paradoxical sensation of warmth and additionally undress. Otherwise, the patients are usually disoriented and exhausted – > exhaustion stage or *adynamia stage.*

Stage 3 – deep hypothermia: core body temperature between 30° and 27 °C, there is a passive increase in muscle rigidity, bradyarrhythmia occurs at the heart, breathing is further depressed to bradypnoea with apnoeic phases. The victims lose consciousness and their reflexes – > *paralysis stage.*

Stage 4 – Vita reducta: Core body temperature < 27 °C, vital functions such as pulse and respiration are further reduced to ventricular fibrillation and respiratory arrest. If vital functions are still preserved, apparent death is present.

The discovery of persons who have died from hypothermia naturally occurs more frequently during the cold season, with hypothermia already threatening at outside temperatures of 10 °C or water temperatures of 20 °C, but under certain circumstances even higher temperatures are sufficient to cause serious hypothermia. People who are particularly at risk are those who are unable to escape exposure to cold due to alcohol, drugs, trauma, internal or psychiatric illness.

Most deaths are found outdoors, but in a good quarter of cases also indoors. Time and again, it can be observed that the corpses are (partially) undressed. In addition, the deceased are occasionally found somewhat hidden (bushes, under a bed or in a cupboard), which is why the suspicion of a sexual offence with concealment of the corpse can arise. However, hiding is an expression of so-called final caving behaviour in hypothermia, which may occur in prolonged agony (Fig. 5.17). This fact must be taken into account when searching for persons suspected of having died from cold.

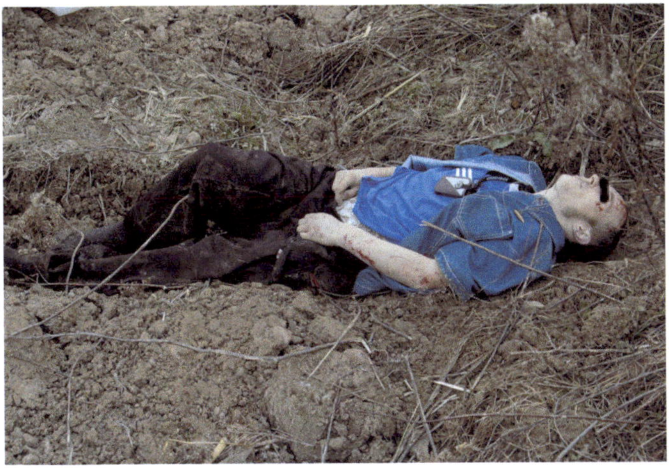

Fig. 5.17 Death from hypothermia in the open. The abrasions on the forearms and forehead are explained by agonal crawling

Morphologically, deaths due to hypothermia show only a few typical findings. The most common is a reddish-brown discoloration of the skin on the knees, occasionally also on the elbows and hips, which is termed cold erythema (Fig. 5.18). The typical internal findings are patchy gastric mucosal hemorrhages (Wischnewski spots) in the sense of erosive stress-induced gastritis and occasionally hemorrhages of the lumbar muscles and autochthonous back muscles. These haemorrhages result from a strong cold tremor, which leads to muscle fibre tears.

5.5.2.2 Frostbite

Similar to burns, frostbite is also divided into stages. Exposure to cold leads to centralization and consequent vascular constriction in the acras (hands < fingers, feet < toes, nose, ears). If this persists over a longer period of time, ischemia of the poorly perfused tissues occurs. This is followed by an inflammatory process that eventually leads to necrosis.

Grade 1 – Due to vascular constriction, the affected area is initially white and numb, then becomes painful and reddened

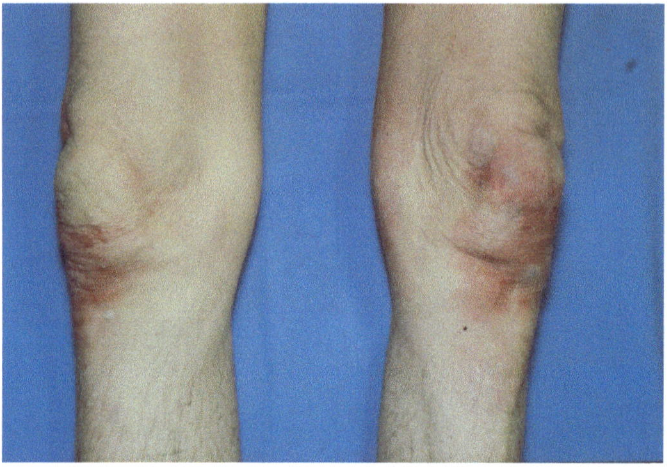

Fig. 5.18 Red discoloration of the knees (cold erythema) is often the only sign of death from hypothermia

(release of histamine-like substances), and can sometimes be very itchy.

Grade 2 – If the area has been exposed to cold for an extended period of time, blistering will occur after rewarming and will be either serous or bloody filled.

Grade 3 – After death of the area turns blue-black. If the patient is "lucky", the necrosis remains dry and does not become infected. If it does become infected, the necrosis is moist and usually smelly.

Special form of frostbite – Similar to frostbite, they occur on the fingers and feet when exposed to cold. However, temperatures below 20 °C can be enough to trigger them. Frostbites are nodular, bluish and watery swellings. They occur particularly frequently on the extensor sides of the fingers and toes. A prerequisite for their development is a congenital change in the vessels.

5.6 Suffocation

Case Histories

You are standing in front of a kebab stand waiting for your well-deserved lunch when a young woman staggers out of the neighbouring house, appearing confused. At first glance, you suspect indulgence from too much alcohol, but when the woman sees you and your vehicle, she approaches you and asks you to help her. You put your kebab aside and go into the RTW with the young woman and your colleague. The presence of another woman seems to be very reassuring for the patient. In the RTW you first notice that the woman's clothes seem to have been put on completely involuntarily, which only increases the confused impression of the woman. She reports that she has woken up in her apartment, lying on the floor, and cannot remember anything. She has severe pain in her throat and swallowing, as if she has a bad sore throat. Your colleague asks the patient to take off her turtleneck sweater and discovers finger-sized hematomas on both sides of her neck. Although the patient is visibly embarrassed, you ask her if she noticed that she had wet herself when she woke up, which she confirms. You suspect a choking attack against the neck with suspected laryngeal fracture. You therefore inform the control centre and take the patient to the nearest larger hospital with an ENT department with the ulterior motive that a forensic pathologist can also be called in there to assess the injuries.

5.6.1 Introduction

Asphyxiation or suffocation is defined as any interruption in the supply, transport or utilization of O_2 between the environment and the body's cells. On the one hand, asphyxiation is a primary cause of death; on the other hand, it is ultimately a component of every dying process at the cellular level. This often makes the forensic diagnosis of death by asphyxiation difficult. Unspecific signs of this are:

Intense, blue-purple hypostasis, hyperemia of the internal organs, a flaccid, anemic spleen, Tardieu spots(petechial hemorrhages of the serous membranes, especially the pleura), and fluid cadaveric blood.

Especially in the field of respiratory distress, there are many medical terms that need to be distinguished from each other:

Hypoxia/anoxia: too little or no oxygen.

Asphyxia: life-threatening interruption of breathing, combination of hypoxia and hypercapnia (increase of CO_2 in the blood).

Dyspnoea: difficult breathing, shortness of breath. In contrast to asphyxia, apnoea – i.e. no breathing – is not a life-threatening condition and hypercapnia or hypoxia need not yet have occurred (e.g. apnoea divers).

Cyanosis: bluish discoloration of the skin and/or mucous membranes due to a reduction in the oxygen content of the blood.

5.6.2 Forms of Suffocation

Because of the different pathophysiological mechanisms, it is advisable to distinguish between internal and external asphyxia, the latter again into atmospheric and mechanical asphyxia. A system of asphyxiation is shown in Graph 5.6.

Atmospheric asphyxiation focuses on the decrease of O_2 concentration in the breathing air. The normal room air concentration of O_2 is 20.9% by volume. If it drops below 17 vol.%, then there are limitations in psychophysical performance. A concentration of less than 15 vol.-% is considered harmful to health, less than 13 vol.-% lethal. Apart from high altitudes (relevant decrease of the O_2-partial pressure from 1600 m above sea level), these are mainly confined spaces without sufficient gas exchange, in which the exhaled CO_2 accumulates. Examples are the plastic bag put over the head as well as containers or trucks in which refugees are illegally transported. Other danger spots are silos, fermentation cellars or well shafts, where CO_2 accumulates because it is heavier than air.

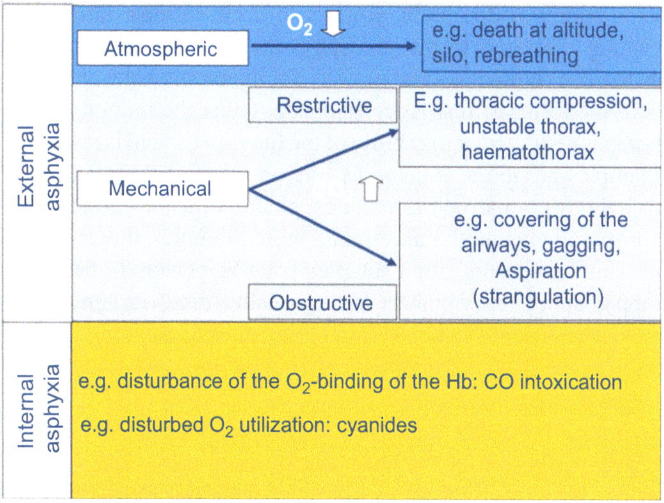

Graph 5.6 External vs internal asphyxia

Since respiratory activity per se is not impaired and CO_2 can be exhaled, there is no feeling of respiratory distress. Rather, a lack of drive and occasionally a mild euphoric mood occur before sudden loss of consciousness.

In mechanical asphyxia, again, two variants can be distinguished, namely a restrictive form and an obstructive form. In both, there is hypercapnia and thus a feeling of breathlessness. A phasic course is typical:

1. Respiratory distress characterized by increased breathing, dyspnea, cyanosis, and loss of consciousness.
2. Asphyxiation spasms, occur due to the lack of O_2 in the brain, accompanied by tachycardia and hypertension, sometimes with urine and fecal discharge.
3. preterminal respiratory pause, respiratory arrest with tachycardia and hypotension
4. terminal respiratory movements/snap breathing

The duration from the onset of asphyxiation to the onset of unconsciousness depends on the mechanism. It is at least 8 s (oxygen reserve of the brain) if there is a complete interruption of the blood supply to the brain, which can occur at most in cases of hanging. In most forms of asphyxiation, both restrictive and obstructive, it takes several minutes for unconsciousness to occur.

In the forms of restrictive asphyxia, either the mobility of the thorax is restricted or the ability of the lungs to expand is restricted. Examples are thoracic compression, an unstable thorax in serial rib fractures or partial rib fractures, pleural effusions or haemato-thorax, and pneumothorax. Among these examples, thoracic compression, as occurs, for example, when a person is buried or trapped under heavy objects that have fallen over, occupies a special position, since not only respiration but also the return flow of blood to the heart, especially in the upper region of influence, is impeded (so-called Perthes' pressure congestion). This results in Dunsung of the face and neck and numerous petechial hemorrhages of the skin of the head, neck, upper chest, and shoulder region. These hemorrhages result from ruptures of skin capillaries overfilled with blood. On the head such congestive hemorrhages are found especially in the eyelids, conjunctiva, and skin behind the ears, but also in the mucous membranes of the mouth and nose. In extreme cases, the entire face is swarmed with petechiae, which is called a "masque ekchymotique".

Obstructive asphyxia is the term used to describe all forms in which obstruction of the airway occurs. These include covering of the airways, gagging, bolusing, aspiration, positional asphyxiation and, to some extent, strangulation.

Covering the respiratory orifices/Smothering is considered to be a low-trace killing method, which, however, only succeeds if the victim is physically far inferior to the perpetrator. This applies to infants, small children or old, frail persons, but also to physically severely disabled people (e.g. in case of quadriplegia) or intoxicated persons. Externally visible are occasional abrasions and drying of the facial skin at and near the breathing orifices, rarely teeth marks and bleeding in the mucous membranes of the mouth. If a pillow or a cloth was used and the victim tried to escape the attack by turning his head away, then the abrasions may be not only scratch-like but also small in area.

Gagging involves inserting foreign materials – often textiles – into the victim's mouth to prevent them from screaming. However, these can swell up in the mouth due to the flow of saliva. When they reach a critical volume of 150–200 ml, the oropharynx is obstructed so that breathing through the nose is no longer possible. If the gag was removed after death, an examination of the victim may still reveal injuries to the oral mucosa and, rarely, textile fibres in the mouth.

Bolus death/Chocking is death by obstruction of the pharynx, usually by large, little to no chewed pieces of food that are too large to swallow and at the same time too large to simply regurgitate. Pressure on the pharyngeal wall causes irritation of the glossopharyngeal and vagus nerves, resulting in bradycardia and orthostatic collapse. The foreign body still remains in the pharynx and obstructs the airway, leading to death by obstructive asphyxia if untreated. Typically affected are people who are alcoholic or who have brain damage, such as Z. n. stroke.

In **aspiration,** the victim inhales foreign material, usually blood or vomited stomach contents. The prerequisite for this is unconsciousness or at least a high degree of clouding of consciousness. Death by drowning is a special form of aspiration (see Sect. 8.6).

Positional asphyxiation/postural asphyxia is the term used to describe all deaths in which the victim is prevented from breathing by a fixed position or unnatural posture.

5.7 Strangulation

Strangulation is an umbrella term for three types of mechanical compression of the soft tissues of the neck, all of which result in hypoxia of the brain. They are *hanging, ligature strangulation*, and *manual strangulation.* All three cause cerebral ischemia by compression of the arteries, asphyxia by squeezing the trachea, and venous congestion by compression of the jugular veins. In addition, there may be a reflex component in all of them due to irritation of the carotid sinus or vagus nerve. How strong this part is, however, depends very much on the individual.

In **hanging,** the compression of the soft parts of the neck is effected by means of a rope tool, which is contracted by the body mass of the victim inside it. The rope tool does not have to be formed into a loop that tightens under tension; an open loop or appropriately shaped solid objects such as a branch fork are also possible. What is essential is the external pressure on the soft tissues of the neck caused by gravity-induced traction of the victim's body mass. Compression of the neck arteries causes a stop in blood flow to the brain. Depending on whether the stop is complete or partial, unconsciousness occurs after a few seconds to a few minutes. If – depending on the snare run and the pressure on the soft tissues of the neck – there is primarily an obstruction of venous return due to compression of the jugular veins, then this also results in a deficiency of blood flow to the brain with unconsciousness, but at a later time than in the case of arterial obstruction. Obstruction of venous return with simultaneous maintenance of arterial inflow leads over time to a cessation of blood flow at the capillary level and thus to an insufficient supply of oxygen to the brain.

In hanging, a distinction is made between typical and atypical hanging: In typical hanging, a running noose runs around the neck in such a way that the lowest point is above the Adam's apple and the highest point (the knot) is central in the neck; the body hangs freely (Fig. 5.19). Contrary to its name, this variant is rare. The more common variant is the atypical hanging, in which the body does not hang freely, no running noose was used or the noose closure is not symmetrical in the neck.

Externally, the victims show a hanging mark corresponding to the course of the snare (Fig. 5.20), often a salivary discharge from the corner of the mouth and – in atypical hanging – punctate haemorrhages of the eyelids and conjunctiva, the skin behind the ears and the mucous membranes of the mouth and nose, up to and including a darkening of the face. The extent of these venous stasis findings depends on the degree of arterial and venous compression. The hanging mark reflects the shape of the strand: if the strand has a round cross-section (e.g., rope), a channel-shaped indentation as wide as the strand will be found. If it has a more rectangular cross-section (e.g. belt, tension belt), then the strand furrow consists of two parallel, narrow, fold-like indentations corresponding to the two edges of the strand tool. Such a hanging

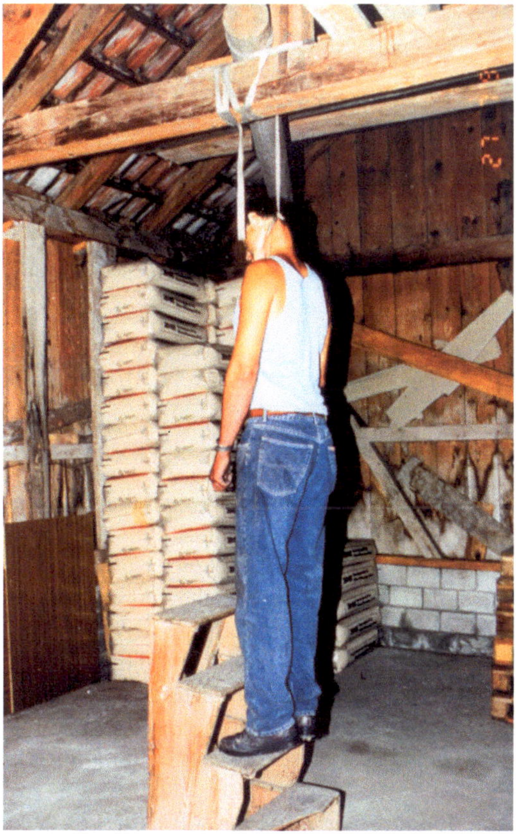

Fig. 5.19 Suicide by hanging in a barn, the hanging point is in the neck, the victim hangs completely free

mark can easily be overlooked. When fresh, the hanging mark impresses as a superficial abrasion, occasionally with small vesicles or skin hemorrhages; with time it dries up and is then easily demarcated. The hanging mark is most indented at its deepest point on the neck, while as it progresses towards the point of suspension it becomes shallower and may also disappear, depending on the shape and course of the loop. On postmortem examination, a compression of the subcutaneous fatty tissue is found under-

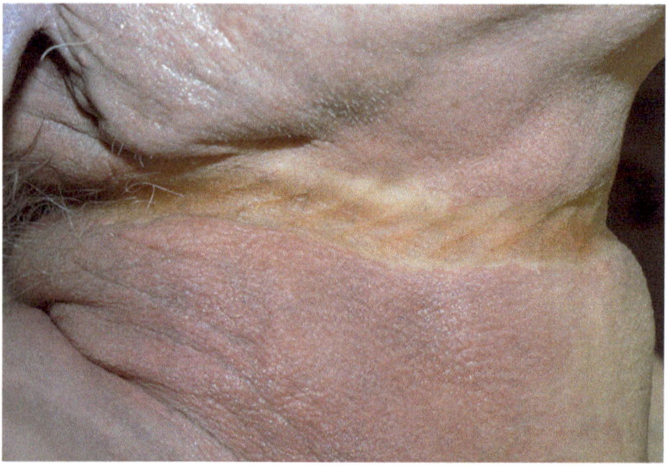

Fig. 5.20 Strangulation mark on the neck after suicide by hanging

neath, but without hemorrhages. Such, on the other hand, is found at the origin of the cervical muscles at the sternum and clavicle. In addition, fractures of the thyroid cartilage horns and hyoid bone may occur, and occasionally tears of the intima of the carotid arteries. Fractures of the cricoid cartilage, on the other hand, are as atypical in hanging as hemorrhages in the other soft tissues of the neck, and should give cause for checking for foreign influence by strangulation.

In **strangulation by ligature**, the soft tissues of the neck are also compressed by a tool, which is, however, pulled tight manually or by machine. Here, as in atypical hanging, there is compression of the carotid and jugular arteries as well as the respiratory tract. However, the vertebral arteries are not compressed, which is why victims often have marked congestive findings on the head: petechial hemorrhages of the eyelids and conjunctiva, facial skin, skin behind the ears, and mucous membranes of the mouth and nose (Fig. 5.21). The ligature mark is usually horizontal, of uniform depth, and circular (Figs. 5.22 and 5.23). However, there are variations depending on the case constellation and the tool. For example, with a soft, wide choke tool such as a scarf, no findings on the neck are to be expected.

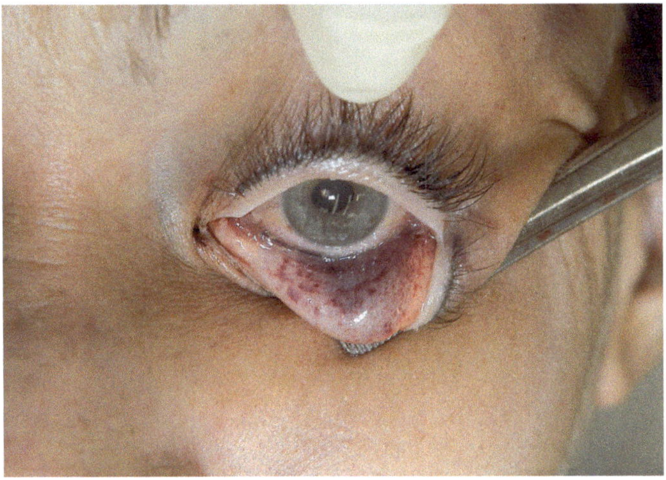

Fig. 5.21 Punctate hemorrhages of the conjunctiva after a fatal strangualtion by ligature

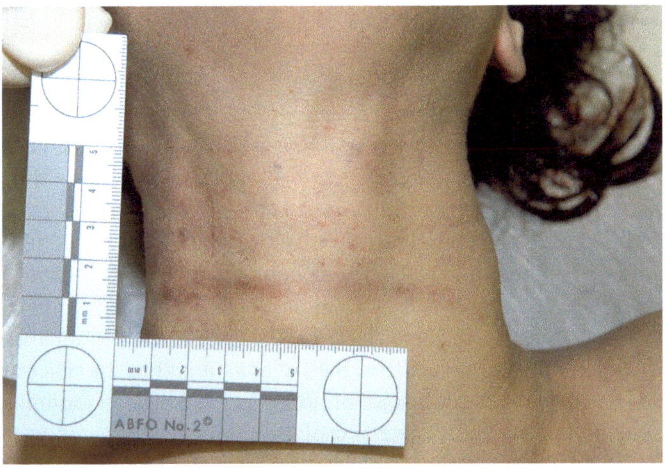

Fig. 5.22 Ligature mark on the neck

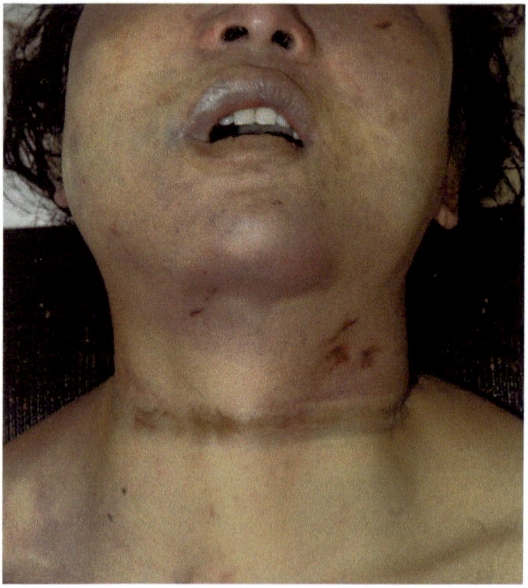

Fig. 5.23 Ligature mark on neck and dunsung and livid discoloration of face as a result of lethal strangulation by ligature

Manual Strangulation does not involve the use of tools in the true sense of the word; compression of the soft tissues of the neck is effected directly by hands, forearm stranglehold or leg scissors. Since in this case there is only limited success in compressing the carotid arteries, unconsciousness results mainly from the combination of venous congestion and compression of the trachea. Therefore, mainly congestion findings on the head are to be expected: punctiform hemorrhages of the eyelids and conjunctiva, of the skin behind the ears, of the facial skin and of the mucous membranes as well as, in case of prolonged venous congestion, a darkening of the face. Congestion of the nasal mucous membranes may lead to nosebleeds. When strangulating with the hands, fingertip-sized haematomas (imprint of fingertips), occasionally merging into one another, and narrow, scratch-like epidermal lesions (abrasions caused by fingernails) can be found on the neck (Fig. 5.24). Strangulation in a headlock (forearm stranglehold) or leg scissors do not result in externally visible changes to the neck (Fig. 5.25). In any case, they are not suitable for assessing a risk

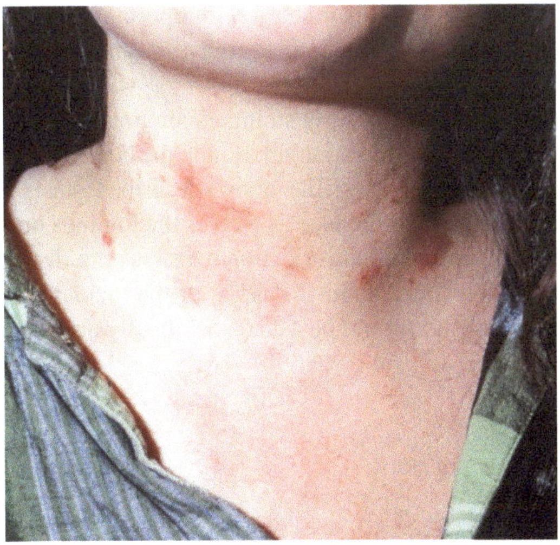

Fig. 5.24 Strangulation marks clearly pronounced on the neck

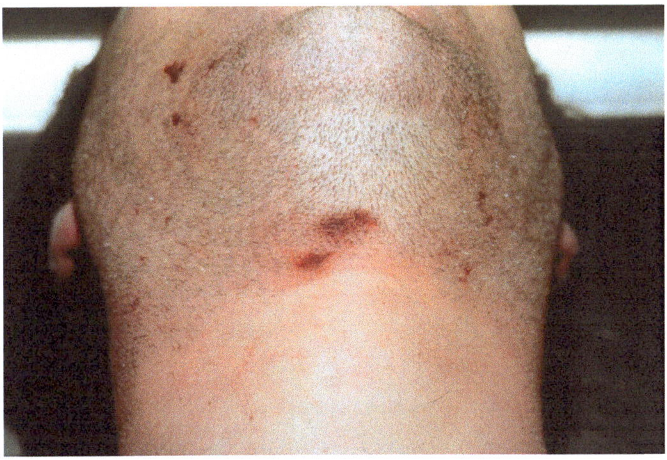

Fig. 5.25 Strangulation marks discretely visible as reddish-brown desiccation on neck and upper jaw

to life. Hematomas and skin hemorrhages on the neck must be considered in a differentiated manner anyway. Not infrequently, so-called love bites are concealed behind the apparent strangulation marks. Therefore, it is much more important to look into the eyelids and conjunctiva and to search for stasis haemorrhages than to look at the neck.

Attacks against the neck by strangers are not necessarily fatal; more common is survived strangulation in the course of a physical altercation. In these cases, the above-described stasis haemorrhages and Dunsung of the face as well as the findings on the neck are also to be expected. Dunsification regresses rapidly, and petechiae can be seen until about 2 days after the incident, occasionally longer. Patients should be asked specifically about:

- Dysphagia
- Hoarseness
- Greyout, seeing stars
- Defecation
- Unconsciousness

6 Traffic Accidents

6.1 Casuistry

You are called as NAW (paramedic team with a doctor onboard) around 23:10 o'clock to a hit person within the city. You find an approx. 40-year-old man lying in a pool of blood with gasping for breath. As it is dark and raining, you decide to crash rescue the obviously polytraumatised patient into the ambulance. You immediately start resuscitation measures as no pulse is palpable and the ECG shows only bradycardic wide complexes. After 25 min of frustrated resuscitation, you pronounce the patient dead. At this time, in front of the ambulance, the police question the driver of the car that hit the now deceased and measure his breath alcohol level, as a clear foetor alcoholicus is noticeable. The driver states that the pedestrian suddenly jumped into the roadway. He still attempted to brake fully, but then hit the pedestrian at an estimated 20 km/h. You look at the accident car with a shattered windscreen with a hole in the upper area, furthermore the bonnet is clearly dented. The injury pattern comes to your mind: The bilateral open lower leg fractures with bone fragments protruding ventrally, the unstable thorax in the dorsal region with visible discontinuity of the thoracic spine and the severe open craniocerebral trauma at the back of the head, together with the vehicle deformation, make you doubt the statements of the driver of the vehicle, since you assume that the pedestrian must have been hit from behind at a

S. Ahne et al., *Forensic aspects in emergency medicine*,
https://doi.org/10.1007/978-3-662-65949-6_6

higher speed. After illuminating the scene of the accident, the traffic police find traces on the pavement which suggest that the passenger car was carried out of a bend due to excessive speed and hit the pedestrian running on the pavement.

6.2 Introduction

Even if internal medical conditions predominate in terms of numbers, traffic accidents are part of the "daily bread" of the emergency medical services. Safety technology in vehicles has improved steadily, but the average speed in road traffic is also increasing. The number of road deaths has steadily decreased, from 11,300 in 1991 to 3046 in 2019 (in Germany), although the number seems to have levelled off between 3000 and 3500 for about 6 years. The number of people injured in accidents, however, has remained persistently high, at about 384,000 in 2019. With trauma centers with standardized equipment available throughout the country, state-of-the-art interdisciplinary trauma care with improved outcomes for the injured has become established. Emergency medical care on site also cannot be compared with that of 30 years ago. Nevertheless, there remains a potential for improvement in trauma care that should not be underestimated. Among other things, and this is the main aim of this chapter, the correlation between accident mechanism and suspected injury pattern is becoming increasingly important in the context of "advanced diagnostics" at the accident site. As an emergency physician, the possible course of the accident at the accident site should be "run through" again in the mind; this not only serves to check the plausibility of the described course of the accident, as in the casuistry of this chapter, but also broadens the diagnostic view with regard to the expected pattern of injury.

In the past, the focus and fixation was solely on the externally visible and unambiguous injuries; today, modern standards of care on site also consider the accident mechanism with its released kinetics in correlation with its potential injury possibilities for this individual case. At the interface to further clinical care, this information is also passed on so that the trauma surgeons can also draw their conclusions from it. And it is precisely in this correlation between accident mechanism and classic trauma sequelae that emergency medicine can learn from forensic medicine, since it is there that all injuries come to light that not infrequently remain hidden to the emergency physician.

The reconstruction of the traffic accident by the investigating authorities primarily serves to clarify the circumstances of the accident. From a legal point of view, the question of guilt and the question of avoidability then arise. These two questions ultimately determine the sentence. Here, medicine can provide important clues, from circumstantial evidence to proof, but here, too, there is a warning against unauthorized investigative activities. It is not the task of emergency physicians to carry out investigations, and certainly not to clarify the question of guilt. After traffic accidents, it is rare for rescue personnel to testify in court. If medical-technical questions arise, a (legal) medical expert is appointed. However, this expert is very dependent on the documentation of the first-aid medical personnel. The medical documents are often the only facts that can ultimately be relied upon.

6.3 Statistics

The following comments are based on data from the Federal Statistical Office for 2018 in Germany.

Accordingly, 2,636,468 traffic accidents were recorded by the police in Germany in 2018, of which 399,293 involved personal injuries. Of these, the majority, namely 328,051 were slightly injured. Just under 68,000 people were seriously injured and 3275 died. Of the accidents involving personal injury, 69% took place in urban areas, 24% rural areas without motorways and 7% on motorways.

These figures should make it clear that traffic accidents, despite the fact that the number of fatalities is fortunately constantly decreasing, continue to be an immense (also economic) problem for our society, which cannot be solved in the medium term by even more sophisticated safety technology. Particularly in the case of two-wheeled vehicles and pedestrians, it is in the nature of things that not much can be improved in terms of safety technology.

Germany ranks in the middle of Europe in terms of the consequences of accidents, which is probably due to the high safety standards laid down, but also to the comparatively high maximum permitted speed. The maximum permitted speed is therefore a permanent subject of political and social discussion. On the one hand, it is a fact that at higher speeds more kinetic energy is released in accidents and the reaction speed is naturally limited. On the other hand, even in countries with comparatively strict speed limits, there are violent accidents in the area of the maximum speed, which make one think of a certain carelessness and a reduced level of attention.

6.4 Classic Accident Scenarios

Typical accidents have their own traumatological laws with a typical injury pattern. Consequently, conclusions about the accident dynamics can also be drawn on the basis of the injury pattern.

In order to present the classic accident sequences, it is useful to distinguish between the following standard scenarios:

- 6.4.1 Cars versus pedestrians
- 6.4.2 Car versus car
- 6.4.3 Car versus two-wheeler

Once you have internalised the basic processes, it is easy for the trained observer to include deviations from these standard scenarios (e.g. fixed obstacle such as a concrete wall or similar) in the considerations. In order to avoid confusion, however, one should initially consider only these three standard situations, with the knowledge in the back of one's mind that in reality it is somewhat more complex.

If there is a lack of plausibility between the accident mechanism and the few visible injuries or even fatal outcome, death from internal causes must always be considered, with the traffic accident as a secondary event. In some accident scenarios, such as hitting a fixed obstacle next to the roadway or steering one's own vehicle into oncoming traffic, suicide is also a possibility.

6.4.1 Cars Versus Pedestrians

In a traffic accident with a pedestrian, the elastic human body absorbs the kinetic energy of the car, which is comparable to a vertical fall of the body onto a hard surface. Therefore, for such accidents, a correlation of speed, fall height and injury severity (for example, as a listing of individual injuries in the Abbreviated Injury Scale – AIS) can also be established and mapped graphically.

In order to understand and reconstruct a concrete accident with all its consequences (damage to the vehicle, injuries to those involved), one must consider the following parameters:

- Contour of the passenger car, especially the shape of the front of the vehicle
- Damage to the vehicle
- Size, constitution and posture of the pedestrian and relationship of the primary point of impact to the body's centre of gravity.
- Type of impact (frontal collision, side impact or grazing the pedastrian)
- Approximate speed of the vehicle at the time of the accident

The pedestrian's clothing must be recovered, even if it had to be cut open for emergency medical reasons (emergency medicine clearly takes precedence over evidence recovery): characteristic traces of the impact of force, such as tyre marks from rolling over or fabric melting at the point of contact, are often visible on the clothing. If the clothing is not left with the police at the scene of the accident, it must be handed over to the hospital with a request for safekeeping, even if it no longer appears usable.

Accidents involving pedestrians are subject to a typical sequence of events in several phases that lead to characteristic injuries. The subdivision into:

- Impact (relation to the body's centre of gravity is important)
- Charging (scooping up) onto the bonnet or knocking over (depending on the centre of gravity of the body and the collision speed)
- Drop

With a little practice, the individual injuries can be assigned to the accident phases.

6.4.1.1 Impact

The primary point of impact of the car with adult pedestrians is usually in the area of the lower leg. The pushing movement caused by the impact often results in characteristic abrasion marks on the soles of the shoes (on both soles in the case of standing pedestrians, on one sole in the case of walking pedestrians). On the skin, marks (e.g. abrasions or bleeding) are to be expected from the contacting vehicle part, usually the front bumper. At the tibia, typical bending fractures occur in a wedge shape (Messerer fracture), with the tip of the wedge pointing in the direction of the force applied. The fracture shape can be used to reconstruct the direction of the impact and also the direction of movement of the pedestrian. The breaking load limit of the tibia is about 20 km/h in young adults and only 5 km/h in older persons. Ankle fractures (typically pilon fractures) are possible due to force transmission of the foot fixed on the ground by the body weight.

6.4.1.2 Scooping-Up

The impact causes an acceleration of the lower legs and an inertia-induced deceleration of the upper body, resulting in a loading onto the bonnet. At the same time, depending on the angle of impact, there is a more or less pronounced rotational movement of the pedestrian about his vertical axis. The impact of the body on the bonnet typically causes an indentation in the front area of the bonnet. Corresponding injuries are hematomas in the area of the hips or buttocks. The head can hit the bonnet (especially in the case of small body size or slow collision speed), the windscreen or, in the case of very large people or higher collision speeds, the upper limit of the windscreen, which regularly leads to a craniocerebral trauma. The damage to the vehicle is not in one line, but is offset from each other, which also allows the walking direction to be reconstructed. The impact of the head often causes the windscreen to shatter, resulting in cuts and splinter adhesions in the wounds. Furthermore, an imprint of the windshield wiper axle on the body is possible, as it is very stable and protrudes vertically from the vehicle. In newer vehicles, the windscreen wiper axle is therefore fitted with a cover. The following rule of thumb for adult pedestrians can provide conclusions about the vehicle speed in relation to the point of impact of the head:

- Up to 40 km/h on the bonnet
- 40–70 km/h in the windscreen
- Approx. 70 km/h in the area of the upper window frame

Only at extremely high speeds above 70 km/h does the victim fly over the passenger car, so that there are only injuries from the primary contact and the drop.

6.4.1.3 Drop

In this final phase, the pedestrian is thrown horizontally or slides off the vehicle at low speed. The energy released during this phase is significantly reduced in relation to the impact with the vehicle, which is why the impact injuries are less severe. Nevertheless, the resulting injuries can mask the primary injuries, making it difficult to differentiate between them. The newly developing injuries are mainly caused by the sliding process on the ground, which not infrequently leads to large and rather superficial abrasions. Another impact, for example against a lamppost, can of course lead to further injuries. The distance between the point of impact and the point of recovery is used to calculate the collision speed.

For this reason, the rescue team should always remember the location of the collision as accurately as possible, even if the patient is quickly transferred to a vehicle for further treatment.

Children are an exception within these three accident phases, as they have a lower centre of gravity and are therefore often not scooped-up and thrown off, but instead pass under the vehicle after the primary impact. Similarly, adult pedestrians are involved in a collision with a truck or rail vehicle due to their near vertical frontal position. Another special case is that of pedestrians entering the interior of the vehicle, which can happen either during the loading phase or when thrown off the vehicle into other road users cars. In this case, the sudden braking and entanglement of the body in the vehicle interior usually results in serious and often fatal injuries.

Other forms of pedestrian accidents include rolling over and being run over. In a run over, the body is parallel to the longitudinal axis of the vehicle. The injuries are caused by the underbody components of the vehicle, and sometimes by clothing getting caught there. In the case of rolling over, the body lies at right angles to the longitudinal axis of the vehicle. The prerequisite in both cases is that the pedestrian is lying on the roadway. This occurs either as a result of the bumping of an upright person by another road user or for other reasons, such as slipping on a slippery surface or falling as a result of higher levels of alcohol. A rollover by the primary striking vehicle is very rare. Much more often it happens due to the following traffic. As a special case, this can also be caused by several vehicles, which of course makes the accident reconstruction much more difficult.

After rolling over, it is not uncommon to find imprints of the tire tread on clothing and skin (Fig. 6.1). The resulting shearing movements of the skin and the underlying soft tissue layers cause stretch cracks in the skin and even decollements of the skin cover from the muscles. Due to the high weight of the vehicle in comparison to the human body, the most severe internal injuries continue to occur. When rolling over the skull, burst fractures and crushing of the skull are possible. Extensive abrasions indicate that the body was dragged a long distance during the rollover or overrun process.

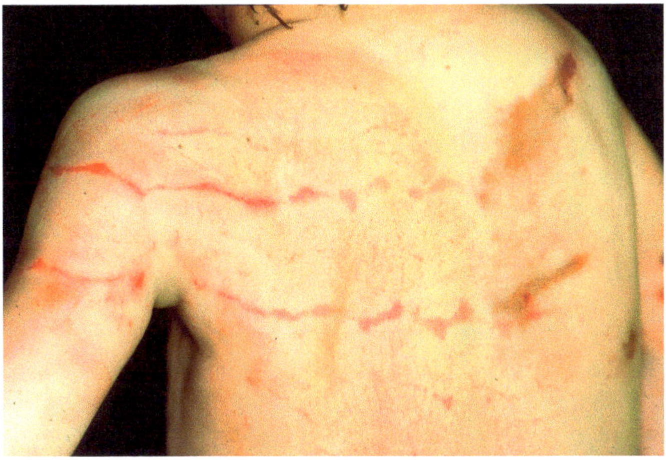

Fig. 6.1 Tire imprint mark on the left shoulder and back of a rolled-over pedestrian

6.4.2 Car Versus Car

In just under 50% of the cases, this is a frontal impact; in the other half of the accidents, the primary impact occurs at the rear or the side.

In the case of a car accident, in addition to the medical care of the injured, a few aspects important for reconstruction should not be lost sight of:

Who sat in which seat?

Particularly important for vehicles with several occupants! Experience shows that it is often difficult to clearly reconstruct the distribution of seats afterwards. Especially if the driver is the one who caused the accident, he has a great interest in concealing his guilt. Not infrequently, it is then claimed that another occupant who died in the accident was the driver. For this reason, it is essential to pay attention to the seating position when recovering the persons and also to note this.

Did you wear your seat belt? Airbag deployed?

Whether or not the seat belt had been worn is a regular question in accident reconstruction and, surprisingly, one that often cannot be answered retrospectively. Belt trauma proves its use, but its absence does not preclude its use, either because there was not much belt loading at all due to the collision (e.g. in side collisions) or because thick-layered clothing alleviated the pressure effect. When rescuing an injured person, it is therefore important to register the state of the seat belt before it is released or cut.

Approximate speed?

6.4.2.1 Front Crash

In a frontal collision, the occupants suddenly and jerkily move forward. Particularly in the case of unbelted occupants, so-called "dashboard injuries" occur with multiple injuries from the knee through the thigh to the pelvis as a result of the transfer and transmission of force on impact with the dashboard (Fig. 6.2). In the

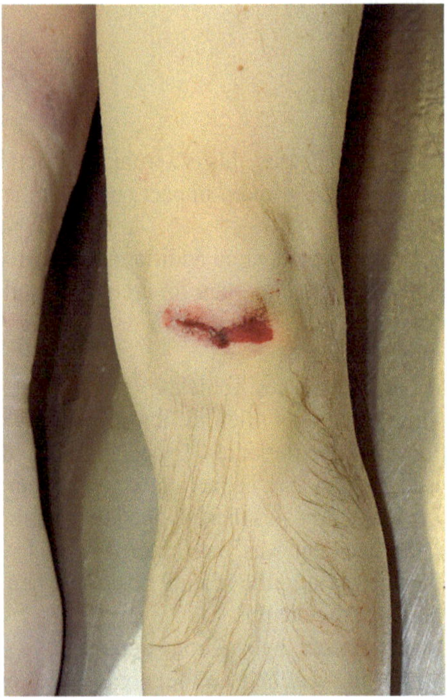

Fig. 6.2 Abrasion of the left knee of a passenger car driver due to impact with the dashboard in a frontal collision

case of reflexive pushing off the ground, ankle fractures are possible due to the muscular fixation of the leg to the ground. Likewise in the case of unbelted occupants, the force exerted on the thorax and abdomen by the steering wheel, dashboard or – in the case of rear-seat occupants – by the backrest is immense, resulting in severe internal injuries, some with only relatively slight external signs. In a frontal impact, there is an extreme pitching motion of the head. This is ***not*** a whiplash injury of the cervical spine as in a rear impact. Especially in case of non-use or technical deficiencies of the seat belt, the head hits the steering wheel or the windshield, a sign for this can be glass splinters in the head wounds. As with the feet, there is often a reflex attempt to support oneself with the hands, but this is no longer successful from an impact speed of 15 km/h and leads to injuries to the forearm and even open dislocation fractures (Fig. 6.3). At higher speeds, serial rib fractures, lung contusions and cardiac contusions up to cardiac ruptures occur. The introduction of modern safety systems, in particular three-point belt and airbags, have led to a considerable reduction in serious injuries, but they cannot prevent them. Some injuries are caused by them in the first place: typical examples are ligamentous haematomas on the thorax and serial rib fractures as well as haematomas on the lower abdomen or in front of the iliac

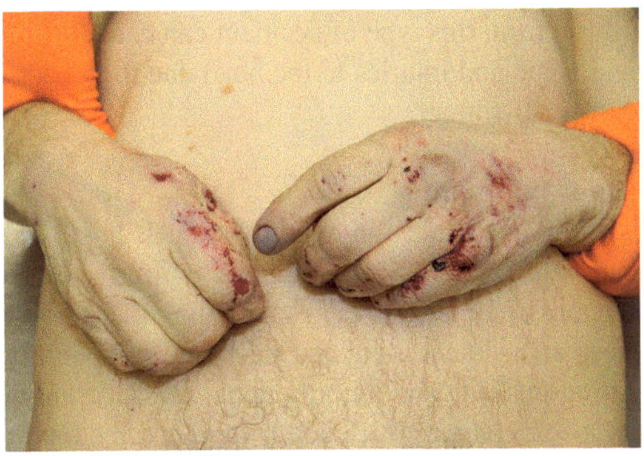

Fig. 6.3 Injuries to hands caused by glass splinters from the windscreen

spines on the pelvis caused by the seat belt. Burns of the hands can occur due to pyrotechnic ignition of the airbags and friction. Since the torso is fixed by the seat belt, there is an even stronger ventral flexion of the head. Belt trauma proves its use, but its absence does not preclude its use. When belt impressions are identified, it is possible to tell whether the occupant was originally seated on the left or right side and whether it was a three-point or two-point belt. In addition, in the event of a frontal collision, additional injuries are of course possible due to objects penetrating the passenger compartment (e.g. engine block).

6.4.2.2 Side Impact

In the case of a side impact, the protective crumple zone is significantly smaller due to the design. More energy is absorbed by the body from the other vehicle entering the passenger compartment, and the seat belt does not provide much protection unless the driver is sitting on the side facing away from the vehicle, where the belt avoids an impact on the inside of the body that is commensurate with the acceleration. Side airbags, on the other hand, are usually very efficient and reduce injury consequences considerably. Nevertheless, the injury severity is higher compared to frontal collisions. Blunt thoracic traumas with rib fractures, haematopneumothorax and lung contusions are particularly common, as are blunt upper abdominal traumas with ruptures of the liver and spleen. The inertia-induced sideways movement of the body resulting from this type of accident can cause distortions of the cervical spine and injuries to the head due to impact with the side window or B-frame.

6.4.2.3 Rear Collision

A classic injury mechanism in rear collisions is hyper-reclination of the head with resulting cervical spine injury (so-called whiplash). There are often legal disputes regarding the causal relationship between an accident event and a cervical spine injury. With a normal sitting position and an orthogonal impact from behind, a minimum speed change of 13 km/h is generally required as a result of the impact. This speed limit is reduced by pre-existing damage to the cervical spine or by an abnormal posture of the cervical spine (so-called out-of-position) at the time of the accident.

Due to the improved safety technology of the current generation of vehicles, there are significantly fewer open injuries than in accidents at the same speed 30 years ago. Nevertheless, a reduction in kinetic energy is by nature only possible to a certain extent. Thus, high-speed accidents with apparent external integrity often result in very serious, even fatal, internal injuries such as rupture of hollow organs or large vessels, since these comparatively heavy organs are only weakly fixed by connective tissue. The higher inertia then finally leads to the avulsion injuries.

If these principles are well understood, they can then also be applied in a modified form to trucks, for example. Another noteworthy special case is accidents involving construction vehicles or vehicles used in agriculture and forestry. Here, crashes can also occur in steep terrain with consecutive rollover movements of the vehicles. It is not uncommon for the occupants to be thrown out of the vehicle because the seat belt is often not fastened.

6.4.3 Car Versus Two-Wheeler

To understand collisions between a two-wheeler and a passenger car, one should distinguish between two basic types:

(a) The car hits the two-wheeler from the side
Initial contact with the car is made with the lower leg, knee or pelvis on the side facing the car. The upper body then hits the bonnet from the side. At higher accident speeds, a rollover movement occurs in the sagittal plane.

(b) The two-wheeler rider collides head-on with the car
The knee joints hit the car first, and then the accident is similar to the pedestrian versus car accident with a scooping up and drop down phase of the two-wheeler rider, only starting from a somewhat higher starting position than with the pedestrian. The traumatological focus here is on thigh and pelvic injuries as well as abdominal, thoracic and craniocerebral traumas caused by the impact with the car. Serious injuries

are often caused by the passenger compartment, which is very stable from the side. The final drop down from the car usually leads to rollover movements in the frontal plane due to the high collision speed. Attempts to support the car regularly result in chain-like injuries to the forearms, elbow and upper arm.

In the case of two-wheeled accidents, the helmet should also always be inspected for damage and then handed over to the police for closer examination. Due to the mostly higher overall speed in addition of the opponents than in the case of a pedestrian collision, there is also a prolonged and intensified final sliding phase, which – unless adequate motorcycle clothing is used – also leads to more serious and larger abrasions.

6.5 Conclusion

In many respects, the rescue service is of outstanding importance here, as it is only possible to assess the forces that have taken place and the accident kinetics on site. Of course, patient care has top priority, but in spite of all the haste, it should not be neglected to visualize the course of the accident from a technical point of view. There is nothing to be said against taking pictures of the accident site in order to present them during the handover to the hospital. Afterwards, however, the pictures should be deleted again immediately and must not find their way into the social media under any circumstances. Even if the initial intention is actually good, this can otherwise lead to serious legal consequences.

Alcohol and Drugs

7

7.1 Casuistry

You are called as an emergency physician to a traffic accident in which a pedestrian has been hit by a car. In addition to hematomas and abrasions, the pedestrian has suffered a fracture of the lower leg. After you have taken care of him, you are asked by the police to take a look at the driver of the car. He has a slightly bleeding contusion wound on his forehead. During the examination you notice the smell of alcohol. The man's answers to your questions are monosyllabic. He seems somewhat absent-minded. The police officers ask you to take a blood sample from the man and to examine him physically with regard to the degree of alcoholisation. However, the car driver refuses the examination. Two days after the incident you are questioned as a witness. The subject of the questioning is, among other things, the question of the extent to which you can say something about the level of intoxication and the driving ability of the accused.

7.2 Alcohol

Alcohol is the most frequently consumed psychogenic substance in Europe. In Germany, the annual drinking quantity per person is 10.5 litres of pure alcohol, which means a daily alcohol intake of

S. Ahne et al., *Forensic aspects in emergency medicine*,
https://doi.org/10.1007/978-3-662-65949-6_7

30 g/d, which corresponds to about three quarters of a litre of beer. At the same time, 7% of the population drink 50% of the amount of alcohol consumed annually. Around 3,000,000 people in Germany abuse alcohol or are dependent on alcohol, that is 5% of adult men and 2% of adult women.

There are numerous ways to come into contact with intoxicated patients in the ambulance service. Examples include:

- Drunk drivers in accidents
- Alcoholised victims in assault offences
- Alcohol-Intoxicated

It is therefore useful and important that emergency physicians and paramedics know the basic pharmacology of alcohol. In addition, the first responders may be questioned as witnesses in subsequent criminal proceedings. The perceptions of medically trained persons in particular play an important role here, as they are able to make statements on the symptoms of drunkenness with more expertise than laypersons. In the case of road traffic offences, this primarily concerns the question of fitness to drive, and in the case of violent offences, the question of culpability.

7.2.1 Pharmacology of Alcohol

With very rare exceptions, alcohol is absorbed into the body by drinking. Other possibilities such as infusions or enemas are rarities in individual cases. Occasionally it is claimed that the alcoholization was caused by inhalation of alcohol vapours or by percutaneous alcohol absorption. These submissions are protective, as no relevant amounts of alcohol enter the body either through respiration or through the skin. The duration of gastric passage is variable and depends on various circumstances in addition to individual factors. A short stomach passage occurs, for example, with drinks containing CO_2 or with an otherwise empty stomach. A long gastric passage occurs when high-proof alcoholic beverages are consumed – especially when larger quantities are involved – or when fatty food has been eaten. The main absorption takes place in the small intestine, although this is not an active process but a passive balancing of concentrations between the intestinal lumen and the bloodstream. Between 10% and 30% of the alcohol drunk does not appear in the blood, for which so-called first-pass mechanisms in the intestinal wall and liver are held responsible. In this case, the alcohol passes directly from the intestine via the mesenteric veins to the liver and is partially broken down there immediately, so that the alcohol then does not appear in the large body circulation at all and thus does not reach the "success organ" brain.

After the alcohol has been absorbed into the bloodstream, it is distributed in all water-containing tissues of the body. Initially, however, there is an imbalance, as the cardiac output (HZV) is not distributed evenly over the entire body. About a quarter of the HZV is available to the brain, which is why relatively high alcohol concentrations occur in the brain during the onset phase. Therefore, more severe psychomotor deficits are observed in this phase than would be expected given the blood alcohol concentration (BAC) determined in the peripheral venous blood. At the same time, the breath alcohol concentration (BAC) is higher than the blood alcohol concentration. Over time, however, diffusion equilibration occurs between all tissues containing water. At this point, alcohol absorption and degradation are in balance, and the peak of the blood alcohol concentration is reached. With "normal" drinking behaviour, this is around the end of drinking. Subsequently, degradation predominates and the blood alcohol concentration decreases.

Alcohol elimination occurs predominantly by enzymatic degradation in the liver, mainly by the enzyme alcohol dehydrogenase. Excretion through sweat, urine or breath is so low that it can be neglected. Degradation is a minimum of 0.1‰, a maximum of 0.2‰, averaging 0.15‰ per hour. Ethanol is the only foreign substance with linear elimination kinetics. Increasing elimination is practically impossible. The occasionally propagated "per-mill-killers" are ineffective.

7.2.2 Alcohol Effects

Ethanol is a substance with multiple effects on the body and mind. It impairs coordination, vision, comprehension, reaction, perception, emotionality as well as circulation, respiration and endocrinium, to name but a few. Even at low concentrations a disinhibition occurs, which is also desired by the users. It facilitates social contacts, increases self-esteem and the subjective feeling of efficiency, increases the willingness to take risks, but at the same time reduces the ability to criticize, the ability to comprehend and the ability to react. Coordination disorders are also noticeable at low concentrations through syllable stumbling, and at increasing levels of alcoholisation through slurred pronunciation and even slurring. In addition, there are movement uncertainties in the sense of ataxias. These also become more conspicuous with increasing alcoholism: unsteadiness of gait, unsteadiness of stance, excessive movements are typical for alcoholics. The effect on the visual organ is noticeable in the form of a restricted peripheral field of vision, tunnel vision, a deterioration in depth acuity, a deterioration in focusing, increased sensitivity to glare with a deterioration in adaptability and – in the case of higher alcohol levels – double vision.

7.2.3 Evidence of Alcoholisation

7.2.3.1 Clinical Picture

In many cases, alcoholization is first noticed by the so-called alcohol odor. However, this does not say much about the degree of alcoholization as it mainly depends on the composition of the accompanying substances (fusel alcohols, aromatic substances) and the duration after consumption. Alcoholic beverages low in accompanying substances, such as vodka, cause virtually no foetor alcoholicus. Other conspicuous features are typical alcohol-related changes in behaviour, motor activity and equilibrium, such as disinhibited, aloof behaviour, slurred speech, swaying when walking and standing, but also rapid mood swings, aggressiveness or tearfulness, to name but a few.

A conclusion from the clinical picture to the blood alcohol concentration is hardly possible. There are many reasons for this: The clinical picture depends on the alcohol habituation of the person concerned, on his other current state of mind (mood, illnesses, injuries), the additional intake of other substances such as drugs or medication and the concrete situation. But also the power of observation and attention of witnesses, i.e. also of persons in the emergency medical services, are individually very different, which repeatedly leads to the fact that the same patient is described in retrospect by one witness as not being intoxicated and by another witness as being drunk. It is much more important to obtain an overview of the remaining psychophysical capacity or the severity of intoxication than to attempt to estimate the blood alcohol concentration.

2.3.2 Breath Alcohol Measurement

The measurement of the breath alcohol concentration (BAC) is an easy-to-use and thus widely used method in the police service to measure the alcoholisation of a person and is therefore also used by police patrols with mobile devices, provided that the person concerned cooperates. There is no obligation for an accused to actively cooperate in the measurement. There is a certain correlation between blood alcohol concentration and breath alcohol concentration, but only in rare ideal cases is there a concentration balance between alveolar air and blood, so that the blood alcohol concentration cannot be reliably determined from the breath alcohol concentration in individual cases. For this reason, there are also different limit values for the breath alcohol concentration and the blood alcohol concentration in road traffic law. In Germany, the measurement of the breath alcohol concentration is only permitted as evidence for administrative offences in road traffic. The limit is 0.25 mg/L alcohol in the breath (§ 24a StVG). A prerequisite, however, is the measurement with an approved, calibrated device for conclusive breath alcohol analysis. Such devices are stationary in the police stations; the mobile handheld devices in the patrol cars are not calibrated.

2.3.3 Blood Alcohol Measurement

The taking of a blood sample requires either the consent of the person concerned or a court order. The blood sample must be taken by a doctor. Alcohol must not be used to disinfect the skin. The police usually provide ready-made blood collection kits, only a dust hose is needed. A protocol to be filled out by a doctor is part of the blood collection. In addition to the personal data of the test person and the time of blood collection, the results of a short, targeted anamnesis and an examination are to be written down or marked in this protocol.

7.3 Drugs and Medication

In addition to alcohol, illicit drugs and medicines are not infrequent causes of road traffic accidents. Depending on the active profile of the substances, disinhibition (e.g. amphetamine, ecstasy, methamphetamine, cocaine) or depressant effects (e.g. cannabis, opiates, benzodiazepines) predominate, which occasionally, but not regularly, can also be inferred from the behaviour of the persons concerned. This is particularly true of the acute state of intoxication with centrally activating substances. These individuals are often conspicuous for their restlessness, urge to move or fluency of speech. On the other hand, a rather tired overall impression with slowing down, dullness of thought, absence or lack of concentration does not automatically indicate a depressant substance. Amphetamines or cocaine initially have a stimulating effect, but after the acute intoxication a phase of fatigue sets in which can last for many hours. It is not possible to conclude from the appearance of an intoxicated person the substance taken, especially since the use of several substances, even substances with opposing effects, is not uncommon.

In terms of clinical appearance, a forensic distinction must be made between uncharacteristic signs of previous drug use and genuine signs of mental deficits that indicate a reduction in physical or mental performance that is relevant to traffic medicine. Uncharacteristic signs of drug influence are, for example: glassy eyes, reddened conjunctivae, shivering or sweating. Indications of impaired driving ability are, in addition to coordination or balance disorders, psychological changes such as poor concentration, prolonged reaction time or reduced comprehension.

7.4 Driving Ability

The following limits for blood alcohol concentration apply in road traffic law (Germany):

0.3‰	Lower limit for the range of relative driving incapacity
0.5‰	Administrative offence according to § 24a StVG (road traffic regulations)
1.1‰	Absolute inability to drive for motorised road users
1.6‰	Absolute inability to drive for cyclists

For relative impaired driving, the blood alcohol concentration must be at least 0.3‰ and there must be additional evidence of an alcohol effect, such as physical signs of failure, driving errors typical of alcohol or an accident typical of alcohol. For absolute impaired driving, the blood alcohol concentration must be 1.1‰ or more; whether additional evidential signs are present is irrelevant.

There are no threshold values for absolute driving incapacity for drugs or medication. According to § 24a para. 2 StVG, an administrative offence is committed if the intoxicating substances tetrahydrocannabinol, morphine, cocaine or benzoylecgonine, amphetamine, MDA, MDE, MDMA (ecstasy) or metamphetamine have been detected in the blood. If, in addition, there are indications of an impairment of performance relevant to traffic medicine, such as physical or mental deficits, driving errors typical of intoxication or accidents, then these prove a drug-related relative inability to drive.

In order to differentiate whether the offence is "only" a misdemeanour or whether the person concerned is relatively unfit to drive, it is essential to know whether or not the person concerned

Table 7.1 Various test procedures

Finger-finger test
Finger-nose test
Cross-eyed test
Horizontal nystagmus
Rotary nystagmus
Romberg test in combination with time perception test
Single leg stand in combination with counting backwards

is showing signs of impairment. In the course of the medical blood test, but also during the police investigation on the spot, the person concerned is therefore offered tests (see Table 7.1), which he does not have to consent to. In addition, an attempt is made to ascertain the mental state of the person concerned, in particular with regard to their ability to concentrate, comprehension and reaction time.

A common plea after alcohol-related road accidents or even questionable drunk driving is post-drunk driving. Here, the driver claims that he or she either consumed all of the alcohol only after the journey or the accident, or at least a large part of it. Here it must be taken into account that a large amount of alcohol can be consumed in a short period of time, but this is accompanied by a pronounced intoxication symptomatology. This can also only occur in the course of a few minutes up to 1 h, which is why attention should be paid to a change in behaviour. It may also be relevant whether empty drinks bottles can be found in the vehicle. The emergency medical team may also be asked such questions at a later stage if the allegation of drunkenness only arises in the course of the investigation or during a court hearing.

There are a number of driving errors as well as road traffic accidents that are typical for intoxicated drivers. "Typical" does not mean that these driving errors or accident constellations only occur when intoxicated, i.e. that they are evidence of alcoholisation or drug influence. However, they do occur more frequently in the group of intoxicated road users than in sober road users.

Typical driving errors include:

- When starting up, people forget to switch on the lights.
- It is driven without putting on the belt.
- There is no dimming in oncoming traffic.
- Direction changes are not displayed or are displayed incorrectly.
- People are driving at very excessive speeds.
- Unclear curves are cut.
- At blind spots, drivers overtake at excessive speed and too close to oncoming traffic.
- Other motorists are denied the right of way.

Typical accidents are:

- Driving straight ahead on (long) left-hand bends
- Patrols of parked or overtaken vehicles
- Rear-end collisions with stationary vehicles (traffic lights, end of traffic jam)
- Collisions with oncoming traffic when turning left

7.5 Capacity to Act and Culpability

In the case of higher degrees of alcoholisation or drug influence, culpability may be considerably impaired or even nullified. The basic prerequisite for a corresponding assessment is that the intoxication is so severe that it is classified as a "pathological mental disorder" within the meaning of section 20 of the Criminal Code in Germany. In order to be able to diagnose such a disorder, it is primarily changes in the behaviour of an accused/defendant that are of interest, rather than the level of the blood alcohol concentration or the blood concentrations of psychoactive substances. Observations and assessments by rescue workers play an important role in the assessment: How capable was the person of acting? Was he able to talk normally or did he slur his words? Was the person still able to walk normally, to move, to perform purposeful and complex movements or were they more ataxic, rudimentary movements? Was the behavior slowed down, was the person mentally absent, or was complex conversation still possible in which differentiated statements could be made and questions meaningfully answered?

In addition to alcohol- or drug-related failure symptoms, the circumstances of the offence and the offender's overall behaviour also play a role. If complex actions can be performed meaningfully over a longer period of time, if adequate reactions to changes in the situation can be made, if longer, meaningful conversations are possible, then this argues against an annulment of the culpability. There is no correlation between the ability to act and culpability in the case of memory lapses (blackouts) that are frequently claimed afterwards. These are often protective claims. Moreover, not remembering what one has experienced does not mean that one was incapable of guilt at the time.

Deaths 8

8.1 Post-mortem Examination

Coroner's inquest is a medical task that is intended to make the following determinations:

- Death occurrence
- Time of death
- Identity
- Cause of death
- Mode of death
- Notifiable diseases

It is regulated in the burial laws and burial ordinances of the different federal states in Germany, which, however, do not differ much in content.

A common mistake is confusing cause of death with mode of death. Cause of death refers to the medical reason for death. The mode of death refers to the circumstances under which someone dies. There are only two possibilities here: Death is the result of disease or the result of violence. In the first case it is a natural

All legal specifications made in this chapter are for Germany!

S. Ahne et al., *Forensic aspects in emergency medicine*,
https://doi.org/10.1007/978-3-662-65949-6_8

death, in the second case a non-natural (= violent) death, whereby one distinguishes here still three sub-forms: In the case of violence by another's hand it is a homicide, in the case of violence by one's own hand it is a suicide, and in all other cases it is an accident. The coroner does not need to make this distinction, much less worry about the legal assessment. What is essential, however, is to recognize an act of violence as the beginning of a causal chain, at the end of which is death. There is no time limit for this causal chain. If the death is ultimately the causal consequence of a traffic accident that occurred years ago, then it is a non-natural death.

Around 900,000 people die in Germany every year. In 96% of cases, this is a natural death as a result of illness. About 38,000 people die a violent death, with about 800 falling victim to a homicide, about 10,000 committing suicide and the rest (about 28,000) dying as a result of an accident.

No additional qualification is prescribed for the post-mortem examination; every practising doctor and doctors in clinics for those who have died in the clinic are obliged to do so. However, there are a few special rules, some of which are regional. The most important special rule is that emergency physicians in most federal states are not obliged to perform a full post-mortem examination, as they can be called out on a new assignment at any time. They can limit themselves to a preliminary post-mortem examination, which serves to establish the death, the time of death and the general condition of the corpse and the external circumstances (e.g. Art. 2 Bavarian Funeral Law). It must be ensured that a complete post-mortem examination is carried out by another doctor. In the case of a new operation, before a certificate has been issued, the family doctor, the medical emergency service or the public health department must be contacted via the operations centre or the police to carry out the post-mortem examination. As a general rule, the treatment of living emergency patients always takes precedence over the performance of a postmortem examination.

A more precise delimitation of the time of death is not the actual task of the coroner, which is why it is sufficient to note the time at which death was ascertained in cases with unobserved onset of death. When resuscitation measures are discontinued, this time is considered to be the time of death.

It is in the nature of things that emergency physicians have to deal with the consequences of violence more frequently than other physicians. It is also in the nature of things that the emergency medical measures in life-threatening conditions are aggressive and invasive, which may lead to overlapping of the original findings on the one hand and to uncertainties in the assessment of the findings on the other, especially if it is not known at the time of the post-mortem examination which iatrogenic injuries were inflicted during resuscitation. It is therefore advisable to leave accesses, drains, cannulae and other measures such as the tube on the corpse and, if necessary, to mark puncture sites with a pen. In the case of unexplained or non-natural deaths, a copy of the (fully completed) emergency medical report should also be given to the police.

In many cases of emergency medical intervention, it is not possible to determine the mode and cause of death. This is due on the one hand to the fact that the patient and his medical history are not known, and on the other hand to the fact that external inspection of the corpse is in very many cases an unsuitable instrument of establishing the mode and cause of death. For example, the absence of obvious injuries on the surface of the body does not at all mean that there was no mechanical violence; intoxication cannot be ruled out externally in any case. In addition, cadaveric appearances may be misinterpreted, discrete injuries may be overlooked, especially under unfavorable examination conditions, late corpse appearances, or poor lighting. In these cases, there is the possibility of indicating an unclear manner of death on the corpse certificate.

If the identity is unclear, the death is due to violence or the mode of death cannot be clarified during the post-mortem examination, then the police or the public prosecutor's office must be notified. The Lower Saxony Funeral Act (§ 4) provides detailed information on the constellations of cases in which this notification must be made (box), which also provides a good guideline for action outside Lower Saxony.

In all cases where the police or public prosecutor's office is notified, changes to the corpse or the place where it was found must be refrained from. This also applies to well-intentioned changes, such as the removal of the tube or cleaning procedures to make the deceased more presentable. In any case, the post-mortem examination must be discontinued as soon as there are indications that the body has been subjected to violence.

The following flowchart is recommended for the performance of the post-mortem examination:

- Death certificate
  - Sure signs of death
  - Note the time of death
- View environment
  - Location
  - Traces of blood, vomit
  - Alcohol, drugs, medications, medical records, weapons, notes …
- Identification
  - Identity card, details of persons present
- Actual postmortem examination
  - Good lighting conditions
  - Undressed corpse
  - Step by step examination from head to toe
  - Inspect body orifices and skin folds
- Consultation with family doctor if necessary
- Termination of the post-mortem examination in the event of indications of non-natural death
- fill out a death certificate
  - Natural death: Transfer to next of kin
  - Non-natural death or unclear mode of death: Handover to police

8.2 Deaths in the Home

When you are called out on an emergency call to a lifeless patient in an apartment, there are three typical scenarios here, namely the case of an expected or at least not entirely unexpected death at home, the case of a completely unexpected death at home, and finally what is referred to in police jargon as an "apartment corpse," namely the case where a person is living alone and the onset of death probably occurred some time ago.

In the first case, it is likely to be an elderly person with pre-existing conditions. Even if the death was not necessarily expected at this time, it is often medically plausible. If you find no evidence of violence to the body at the post-mortem examination, if you have been able to form a coherent picture of the medical history after consulting the family doctor, and if the circumstances you now find do not give you an uneasy feeling, then there is nothing to prevent you from certifying a natural death, provided you carry out a full post-mortem examination.

The second case typically involves a person of middle to advanced age, with no known pre-existing conditions, where the onset of death was sudden and unexpected for the relatives. While this does not rule out illness as the cause of death, actively naming it is pure speculation. Even the family doctor, who may have been contacted, is usually unable to help in such a case, as he is just as perplexed and does not know anything relevant to report from the medical history. In such a case, it is advisable to certify an unclear mode of death and to inform the police. The police must be informed all the more if the circumstances of the discovery of the corpse make one think of an accident or some other kind of violence. It is not at all uncommon for relatives to have altered the situation, for example to cover up an auto-erotic accident or a suicide.

8.3 Road Traffic Fatalities

Road traffic accidents are among the most frequent emergency medical interventions. Occasionally, the injuries are so severe that it is not possible to stabilize the victims on site, so that death must be determined after frustrated resuscitation. As a rule, these are polytrauma or isolated craniocerebral trauma. Occasionally, but rarely overall, it only appears to be an accident, but is in fact a natural death in road traffic or a suicide. This distinction can hardly be made with certainty at the scene, even if it is occasionally suspected – because of the then rather mild accident damage to the vehicles. In the case of deaths in road traffic, it should generally be assumed that the death was not of natural causes. The police, who should be notified, are usually involved anyway. Further information on this subject can be found in Chap. 6 (Road traffic accidents).

8.4 Railway Fatalities

As with road traffic accidents, emergency medical interventions on railway lines are not uncommon, whereby contact between a train and a person is not necessarily fatal, but is usually accompanied by very serious injuries. From a criminal justice perspective, suicides dominate fatalities, followed by accidents. The Federal Railway Authority lists the respective figures in its annual reports; they range between 700 and 900 cases per year. The number of people killed in accidents has been between 146 and 179 per year over the last 10 years.

Suicides on railways are usually carried out in such a way that the victims are on the tracks and allow themselves to be run over by the approaching train in an upright, sitting or lying position. Some do not go onto the track until just before the train is approaching, to ensure that the driver cannot bring the train to a halt before then. In other cases, the suicides place their necks on the tracks so that they are decapitated by the train. Whereas in the cases by running over the body is irregularly crushed, in the case of decapitation it is comparatively intact, as the body often lies outside the track bed.

At the post-mortem examination, the external impact of force and thus the non-natural death is obvious. Particular attention should be paid to whether injuries are visible that cannot be explained by a train passing over the body. It is also advisable to pay attention to the appearance of death marks. In the early phase after the onset of death – and thus the period in which emergency medical intervention on the track typically takes place – they are only sparsely pronounced anyway. However, they will not be able to develop to normal strength even in the course of the next few hours due to extensive external blood loss. Therefore, strongly formed hypostasis on a crushed body are to be regarded as an indication that death has already occurred temporally some hours before the overrun. In this case, the suspicion is that it is a homicide that the perpetrator wanted to dissimulate as a suicide by placing the body of the deceased on the rails.

8.5 Deaths in Places Open to the Public

From a criminological point of view, deaths in places open to the public are linked from the outset to the possibility of outside influence or an accident, which is why it is advisable to certify at least an unclear mode of death. For the emergency physician, there are also the usual difficulties that no medical history is known and, in addition, that the identity is often unclear. In any case, the possibilities of a thorough post-mortem examination are not given in public. Depending on the circumstances, it is advisable to carry out a post-mortem examination initially only for orientation purposes, preferably together with the criminal investigation department, and if necessary to dispense with an on-site post-mortem examination altogether. If necessary, it can be carried out in detail in a place protected from prying eyes (mortuary at the cemetery, funeral home), if this offers sufficient lighting conditions. The advantage of a second, delayed postmortem examination is that some findings are better demarcated than in the very early postmortem phase. In older forensic literature, the value of a second post-mortem examination was repeatedly emphasized, since, for example, skin desiccation following abrasions, but also hematomas, are more clearly visible during this examination than shortly after death.

8.6 Death in Water

Deaths in water are not necessarily deaths by drowning, even though this is statistically the most common cause of death in this group of cases. In addition to drowning, which can be divided into two subtypes (typical drowning vs. abbreviated drowning), it can also be a so-called bathing death, a death from natural causes that occurs accidentally in the water, or an otherwise traumatic death. Finally, there is also the possibility that the death occurred on land and the body was taken into the water.

Drowning is the result of inhalation of water (or another liquid) and thus a particular form of aspiration, i.e. suffocation due to obstruction of the airways. Two variants are distinguished, which also differ in the pattern of findings. The typical drowning occurs in stages: After reflex inspiration, there is voluntary cessation of breathing (apnea stage), followed by the dyspnea stage of varying duration, in which there is repeated aspiration of drowning fluid, coughing attacks, and holding of breath until tonic-clonic convulsions then occur due to progressive hypoxia (convulsion stage), and finally, after a terminal respiratory pause and final gasping breath, death occurs by respiratory paralysis. The drowning process can last for many minutes depending on the physical condition.

The only external sign of a typical drowning death is the discharge of fine-bubbled, whitish froth from the respiratory orifices; a finding that is particularly noticeable immediately after the body has been retrieved from the water, whereas it becomes less and less pronounced in the course of the following hours as the froth decomposes (Fig. 8.1). The froth is the result of the dyspnoea stage: the inhaled water mixes with air and mucus from the bronchial glands during the breaths and coughing attacks, which – similar to the asthma attack – leads to obstruction of the airways.

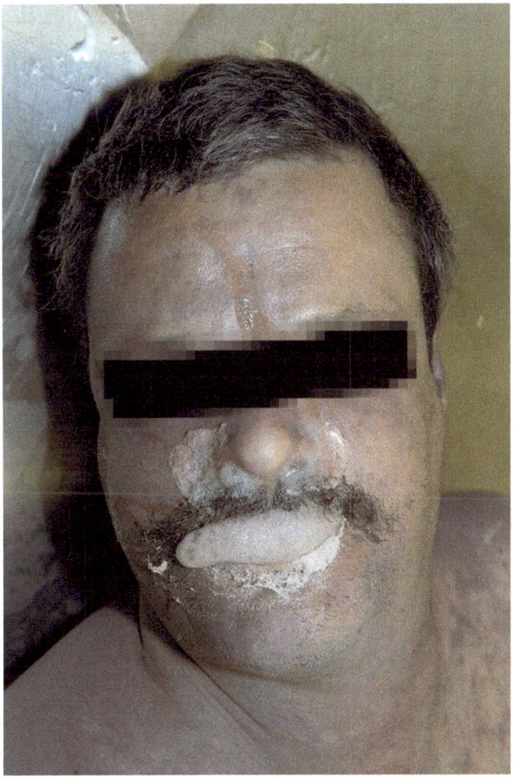

Fig. 8.1 Particularly shortly after recovery from the water, a plume of froth in front of the respiratory openings can be indicative of the cause of death, especially in the case of corpses that have not undergone much decay

In abbreviated drowning, the victim gets under water in an unconscious state with the respiratory openings, which means that the resistance to inhalation of water and thus the stages of apnoea and dyspnoea are absent. In these cases, the plume of froth in front of the respiratory openings is also absent. Externally suggestive in individual cases may be injuries to the scalp, suggestive of blunt trauma to the head with subsequent unconsciousness. In the case of other causes of unconsciousness, such as intoxication, such indications are naturally absent.

Autoptically, in cases of death by typical drowning, in addition to the froth in the respiratory tract already mentioned, one finds a strongly marked, dry pulmonary distension (emphysema acquosum) (Fig. 8.2) with blotchy, washed-out hemorrhages in the visceral pleura (Paltauf's spots), watery fluid in the stomach, and in prolonged drownings also in the upper small intestine, a reddish discoloration of the intima in the great circulation as a result of hemolysis, and fluid in the paranasal sinuses (Svechinkov's sign). Hyperexpansion of the gastric inlet, which may occur when

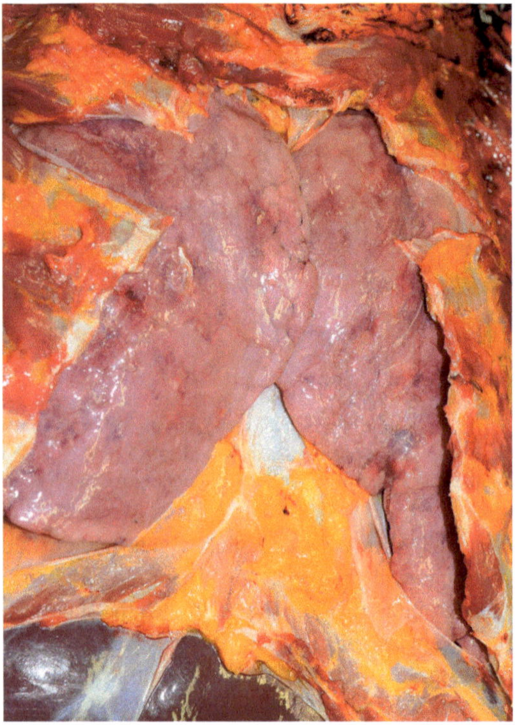

Fig. 8.2 Internal drowning finding: dry lung distension due to obstruction of the airways by froth, mucus and water. Here the leading edges of both lungs overlap

swallowing large amounts of fluid and may lead to tearing of the mucosa (Fritz's sign), is another finding, albeit a very rare one.

So-called bathing death is a reflex-mediated death that cannot be proven autoptically. Cold water in particular can lead to vagal syncope (e.g. Ebbecke reflex, nasal mucous membrane reflex) due to irritation of the trigeminal nerve, as a result of which the affected person faints and therefore becomes submerged with the respiratory orifices. As in abbreviated drowning, inhalation of water then occurs without resistance, which is why the classic autoptic drowning findings are absent. These reflexes are particularly strong in infancy, which may explain why young children drown in a shallow puddle even if they are only face down in it.

In many cases, deaths in water are only discovered and recovered after a few days. By this time, the above-mentioned findings, which are in any case sparse during external post-mortem examinations, are usually obscured by putrefactive changes in the body. In addition, prolonged exposure to water leads to the formation of the waterlogged skin also called washer womans skin (Fig. 8.3), a wrinkled, whitish swelling of the skin of the groin on the palms of

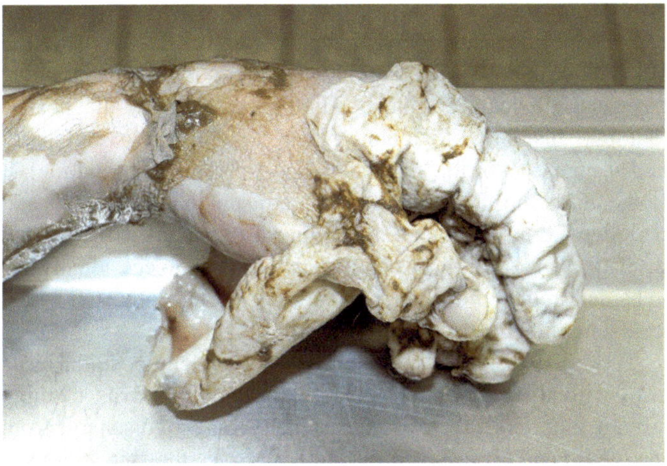

Fig. 8.3 Waterlogged skin: Wrinkling of the skin on the hands. The epidermis can be partially peeled off like a glove during prolonged immersion in water

the hands and soles of the feet. In the case of corpses found in flowing waters, post-mortem injuries may result from dragging the body over the bottom of the water or obstacles. In waters with boat traffic, injuries may result from the body being caught by the propellers as it passes over. Protective grids are installed in front of locks or weirs with turbines to prevent flotsam from entering. These grids are regularly cleaned by dredgers with grab arms. If there was a human body in the flotsam, it can also suffer injuries from the grab arms during recovery.

8.7 Death in Infancy and Childhood

Childhood deaths are among the most emotionally stressful in emergency medical service. The focus is not on the medical management of the emergency situation, but on the drama of this hardly comprehensible stroke of fate. It is therefore all the more important to keep a cool head and not let emotions get the better of you.

"Sudden infant death syndrome" (synonym: sudden infant death syndrome, cot death syndrome, SID, SIDS) is the sudden and unexpected death of an apparently healthy infant between the 8th and 365th day of life, in which it is not possible to determine the cause of death despite maximum post-mortem diagnostics (autopsy, histology, toxicology, bacteriology, analysis of pregnancy, course of birth, "medical history" and finding situation). It is the third most common cause of death in the postneonatal period in Germany – and it is a diagnosis of exclusion that cannot be made at all on site. The death of an infant, as it occasionally has to be determined in the field, is therefore not to be equated with a "sudden infant death".

Typically, the infant is found dead in a prone position in its crib, with its head under a blanket or pillow and its clothing sweaty. Externally, there are occasionally traces of discharge from the mouth and nose or vomit (Fig. 8.4). Since the skin still has a thin, tender horny layer, desiccation of the facial skin or lips is a frequent finding, which is often misinterpreted as evidence of mechanical violence (Fig. 8.5). Occasionally, single petechial

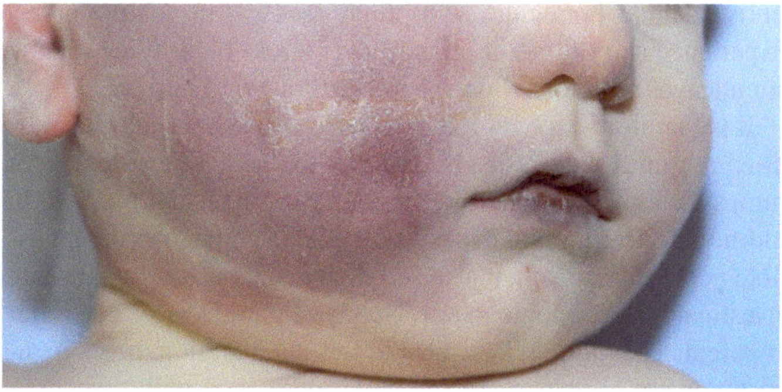

Fig. 8.4 Fluid draining from the nostrils and incipient desiccation of the labial red in sudden infant death syndrome

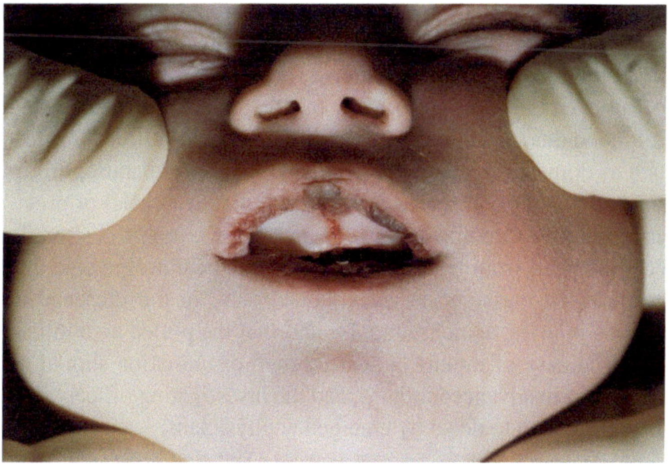

Fig. 8.5 Postmortem artifact in SIDS: desiccation of the lip red and the upper lip frenulum

haemorrhages of the eyelids and conjunctiva may also be seen. These are consequences of upper influence congestion, for which there may be many causes. Generally, again, petechial haemorrhages are indicative of an attack against the neck or compression of the chest until proved otherwise. In fact, infant deaths consistently include homicides – as high as 15% in some studies. Experience shows that in infancy, even gross blunt force trauma often leaves no or only non-specific external findings.

It is therefore strongly recommended that such deaths be classified as "unexplained death" and that the police be notified. An autopsy is equally strongly recommended for several reasons. In addition to determining the cause of death and uncovering a possible non-natural death, it also serves to exonerate the parents and investigate the phenomenon of "Sudden Infant Death." The relief of parents is an important aspect in this enumeration. It is a natural reflex for parents to blame themselves, feel guilt, and have difficulty getting over the death of their child. Experience and numerous studies show that it is relieving for parents to be told that they did nothing wrong and that the death was a fateful event. There is no obligation to perform an autopsy on children in Germany, with the exception of the Federal State of Bremen (§ 12 Bremen Law on Mortuary Matters).

But even beyond the first year of life, sudden and unexpected childhood deaths can occur. There are many possibilities for this, such as domestic accidents, accidents at play, child abuse, fulminant inflammatory diseases (e.g. pneumonia, urosepsis) or previously unknown malformations. In these cases, too, it is strongly recommended from both a forensic and medical perspective that the death be classified as unexplained – or, in the presence of obvious injuries, as non-natural – and that the police be notified. As in the case of infants, a post-mortem examination should be carried out in advanced infancy, and the investigating officers may also be advised to do so by emergency physicians.

Abuse Offences 9

9.1 Harms to the Body

According to § 223 StGB (german criminal code), bodily harm is physical abuse or damage to health. Physical abuse is defined as a nasty, inappropriate treatment, whereby the victim is not insignificantly impaired in his physical well-being or physical integrity. Whether or not this causes pain, and to what degree, is irrelevant. Harm to health is the causing or increasing of a pathological condition, for example by the sale of spoiled food. The bodily harm is further differentiated into a dangerous bodily harm (§ 224 StGB) and the serious bodily harm (§ 226 StGB). Simplified, § 224 applies if a weapon/dangerous tool was used for the act, and § 226 if the bodily harm causes serious permanent physical damage, such as blindness, the loss of a limb or a permanent disability. The degree of penalty ranges from 3 months to 10 years imprisonment.

9.2 Domestic Violence

Domestic violence can be perpetrated in any way, emotionally/psychologically, sexually or physically and of course in combination. It does not matter whether the partners are married, cohabitat or "just" live together. The location of the act is also irrelevant,

S. Ahne et al., *Forensic aspects in emergency medicine*,
https://doi.org/10.1007/978-3-662-65949-6_9

what matters is that the perpetrator and victim are in a relationship with each other. These acts are often accompanied by shame on the part of the victim and are not infrequently denied or attributed to an accident or oversight. Children are to be particularly protected in this context. Even if they themselves may not be victims of violence because, for example, the wife beats the husband but is a loving mother to the children, they are nevertheless also victims and must not be forgotten in the treatment. They are emotionally burdened and in addition they "learn" that problems are solved with violence, which they may implement themselves in adulthood without regulatory intervention.

Special Form of Elder Abuse

Especially the ambulance service is confronted in a multitude of cases with elderly patients in the most different situations. Unfortunately, there is also violence against elderly patients, who are usually physically inferior and, in the case of dementia, are also unable to report an act against them. A motivation for violence up to the killing of elderly people can be financial dependencies, an excessive demand by the nursing situation, but also sexual needs in case of sexualized violence mostly against elderly women.

In order to identify possible elder abuse or neglect, attention should also be paid to accurate documentation, especially if restraint measures have been used and may have harmed the patient. Signs of neglect also need to be documented. Patients are often no longer able to defend themselves, which makes it all the more necessary to have people from the outside looking out for their best interests.

9.3 Sexual Offences

9.3.1 Casuistry

In the evening hours, you are requested by the police as the crew of an emergency ambulance to a middle-class residential area with multi-family houses – you are given the keyword "domestic violence". In the midst of three patrol car crews, you find a 34-year-old woman who appears intimidated and who states that she has been beaten by her husband (and father of her three children aged 2, 5 and 7) in the course of an argument. The woman makes a stressed and in the next moment apathetic impression. She says to you that she does not want a more extensive examination or hospitalization, she had only asked for a doctor to escape the questions of the police officers. You ask the woman to allow you to see her injuries, at least in an orienting manner. In addition to a swelling of the upper lip, the patient shows you several pinpoint hematomas on the insides of her upper arms. There is a discrepancy for you between the minor injuries and the mental state of the woman. Thereupon you ask the police officers for an undisturbed examination possibility in the bedroom of the flat. There, asked again about the injuries, the patient bursts into tears and states that she had been raped by her husband. She hopes that you will leave her alone soon, because she does not want to press charges and she reminds you of your duty of confidentiality. She does not want the children to know about the rape. After a longer conversation with the offer of help to present the woman to a gynaecological outpatient clinic, she agrees on the condition that she first organises care for the children and that a friend is allowed to accompany her. She adds that due to the organisational effort it might not be possible to visit the clinic until the following day. Now she wants to freshen up and put on new clothes before meeting the children.

Once again you urge the woman to file a criminal complaint, also in the interest of her children, and advise her to go to a clinic as soon as possible for a more detailed examination and documentation of the findings, irrespective of any possible criminal complaint. For an adequate securing of evidence she should neither wash herself nor change her clothes, even if this was unpleasant for her.

You then inform the police, in agreement with the patient, that she had agreed on an examination in a clinic after child care had been provided. You say that the patient asks for time to think about possible criminal charges against the man taken into custody by the police.

9.3.2 Introduction

This chapter deals with alleged victims of a sexual offence or, as the legislature puts it, “offences against sexual self-determination” in the sense of:

§ 174a Sexual abuse of prisoners, persons in custody of the authorities or sick persons and persons in need of assistance in institutions
§ 174b Sexual abuse using an official position
§ 174c Sexual abuse taking advantage of a counselling, treatment or care relationship
§ 177 Sexual assault; rape
§ 178 Sexual assault and rape resulting in death

A separate section is devoted to the sexual abuse of children (§ 176) in the chapter on child abuse (Sect. 9.4). Therefore, the corresponding special aspects are missing here. Nevertheless, the content of this chapter can also be applied to children to the greatest possible extent.

A rescue service call due to a sexual offence that has taken place is not very common, yet a profound knowledge of the necessary procedure is important in order to increase the chances of solving the crime. Usually, there are no witnesses to the crime and the physical signs are often weak. An adequate and thorough examination and evidence recovery by an investigator who is experienced in the best case scenario are therefore often essential for a conviction. Certainly, these measures are not the task of the emergency medical service, but the emergency doctor or the rescue service personnel should nevertheless set the necessary course quickly and purposefully.

The highest priority in dealing with the victim of a sexual offence is an empathetic appearance and action. The victim’s sense of shame must be respected at all costs.

9.3.3 Statistics

The following information relates to the Police Crime Statistics 2019 for Germany and of these only the attempted as well as completed cases of sections 174, 177 and 178.

The police in Germany became aware of 15,929 cases, of which 87.7% were solved, 12,965 perpetrators were recorded, of which 96.8% were men. 81.5% of the perpetrators were over 21 years old, 7.4% 18–21 years old, 9.5% 14–18 years old, 2.4% under 14 years old. 20.86% of the perpetrators were non-German citizens. The police crime statistics recorded 15,697 victims, 87.6% of whom were female.

Unfortunately, we know that the number of unreported cases is many times higher. Often, criminal charges are not filed because the victim and the perpetrator know each other well or are related to each other and the victims are afraid that filing criminal charges will damage the family even more than is already the case. But even in the case of unknown perpetrators, it is not uncommon for the police not to be informed due to unfounded shame.

9.3.4 Versions

The legal classification of "offences against sexual self-determination" summarises the commonality of the many different types and forms of sexual offences.

The term rape is usually equated with penetration or at least the external touching of the sexual organs. If this does not happen, one speaks of sexual assault.

Sexual assault is when the victim is forced to perform sexual acts on the perpetrator.

Many perpetrators experience sexual arousal or satisfaction through their actions. However, there are also perpetrators for whom gaining or asserting power or humiliating the victim is the focus of their interest. Often there are similar events in the history of the offender, but in the victim role.

9.3.5 Diagnostics

9.3.5.1 Questioning

The questioning for the exact reconstruction of the crime is the task and privilege of the police. The examining physician limits himself to those questions that have relevance and consequences for his diagnostic measures. This includes:

Where was the crime scene (apartment, forest, etc. because of clinging traces)?
How long ago was the crime committed (time of the crime)?
What was the nature of the violence?
Are there any physical complaints?
Was a condom used?
Did vaginal and/or anal and/or oral intercourse occur?
Where was ejaculated?
Was there any violence to the neck?
When and with whom (later perpetrator?) was the last voluntary sexual intercourse?
When was the last menstrual period or are you taking contraceptives?
Are there any pre-existing diseases or injuries in the anogenital area?
What was the behavior after the crime (body cleaning, change of clothes)?

If the victim provides information on the course of events, this information shall be reproduced in the words of the victim in the further course of the documentation.

Through the questioning, it is also important to determine whether there was any mental impairment at the time of the crime. Was the victim under the influence of medication, alcohol or drugs? Is there any evidence of a psychiatric illness or mental retardation in the medical history?

9.3.5.2 Investigation

The physical examination must take place as soon as possible after the crime, so that no traces are lost or discreet injuries can still be proven. To this end, it is also important to convince the victim, contrary to the frequently expressed wish, not to attempt to clean their body or change their clothes. Even though this can be very stressful for the victim, it is very important for the search for evidence.

The examination must take place in a comfortable and materially adequate condition, including a gynaecological examination chair. The necessary material must be available and ready to hand. A calm and professional atmosphere with a maximum of empathy is very important. The sense of shame must be preserved and, not least for this reason, duplicate examinations should be avoided. Therefore, the physical examination and forensic examination should be done at the same time. If possible, the examiner should not be alone with the alleged victim; if it is somehow feasible, a woman should be present. At the beginning, the clothing should also be documented in order to be able to prove later whether a change of clothing has taken place before.

The extent of the examination is to be discussed with the victim, if desired, individual aspects of the examination can also be waived with the risk of not discovering all findings. Of course, strict observance of the duty of confidentiality must be ensured, and the results of the examination may only be passed on after the victim has released him or her from this duty. The situation is only different if the investigating authorities order an examination because, for example, the alleged victim could also be the perpetrator. In such a case, there is an obligation to conduct a full-body examination and there is no duty of confidentiality vis-à-vis the investigating authorities with regard to findings that are connected with the crime. However, there is a right to refuse to testify if, for example, the victim is related to the perpetrator.

In a later court hearing, it is very important to relate the findings to the course of events described by the victim or the suspect, or to interpret discrepancies correctly. However, this is the task of the court and not of the examining physician. The forensically inexperienced physician in particular must limit himself to a purely descriptive reproduction of his findings, an interpretation of which can then be made by the court through a forensic pathologist appointed as an expert. The precise assessment of the injuries is particularly important if the perpetrator comes from the victim's immediate social environment (this is the case in 60–80% of cases) and claims that the sexual act was voluntary.

For the exact appearance and description of the possible injuries, please refer to the dedicated chapters of this book, such as on blunt force. Nevertheless, in connection with sexual offenses note the following features of the physical examination:

The absence of injuries does not exclude a crime, nevertheless, with careful examination, morphological changes can be detected in 70–80%. Especially in the absence of physical resistance (for example, due to a threat with a weapon), the findings may also be very subtle and detectable only for a relatively short time.

Care must be taken to document all findings accurately, even if the individual injuries do not require treatment. Writing down "multiple haematomas" or "contusions" without specifying whether there is an abrasion, haematoma or similar does not make sense, as this information is not to bc used. Particular attention should be paid to formed injuries (bite injury, ravishment, strangulation marks, defensive injury, and injuries to the wrists, upper arms, and inner thighs) (Figs. 9.1 and 9.2). In addition to the written description of the findings, photographic documentation is indispensable, which must always be carried out with a scale and under good lighting conditions, as this is the only way in which findings that may be difficult to recognise can be easily depicted and reproduced.

Two special cases are the use of force against the neck and the abutment injury:

If there is anamnestic evidence of a violent attack on the neck, petechiae on the conjunctiva and the face should be observed in addition to the possible grip marks, as they may indicate an increased tissue pressure as they occur in the context of a choking attack.

Especially in the case of sexual offences, it is not uncommon for abutment injuries to occur at the lying-in places, which may

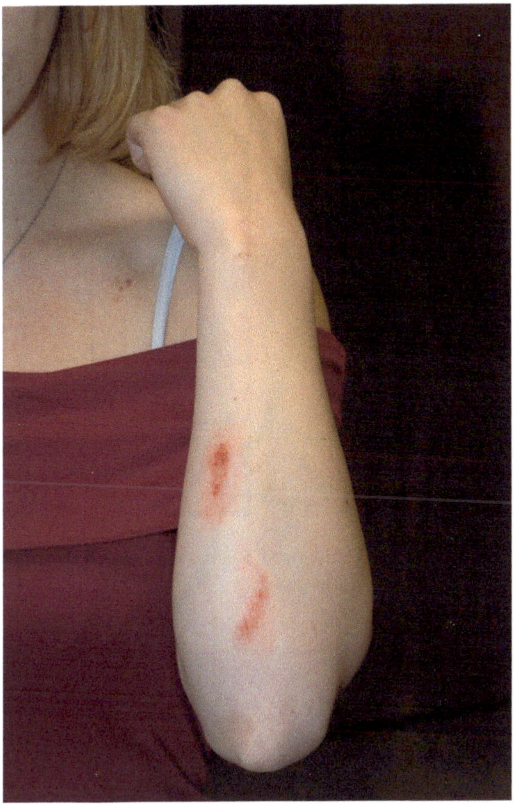

Fig. 9.1 Abrasions following blunt force trauma to the ulnar side of the left forearm. Typical localization for defensive injuries

reflect indications of the body posture and the use of force during the offence (Fig. 9.3). Furthermore, scratch marks on the chest, hips and buttocks may result from forcible undressing.

9.3.5.3 Trace Evidence/Laboratory Diagnostics

The securing of evidence is of great importance in sexual offences, as there are usually no witnesses to the offence and the offence can only be proven by a valid set of traces. Even if they are not carried out in the rescue service but in the gynaecological clinic or

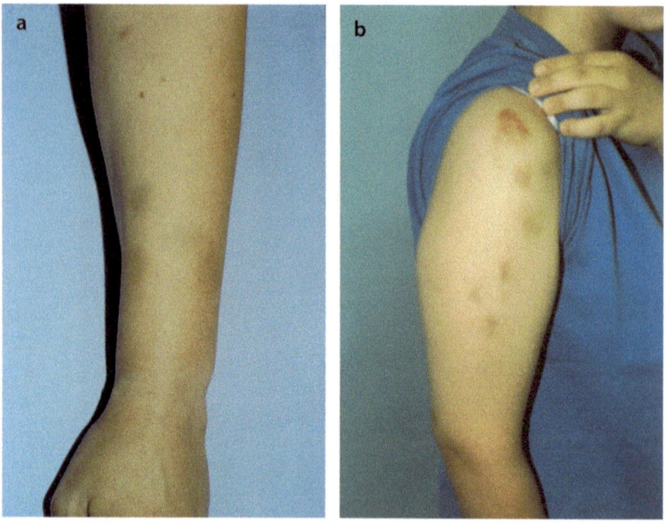

Fig. 9.2 Grip marks: fingertip-sized haematomas on the forearm (**a**) and upper arm (**b**) as a result of firm gripping

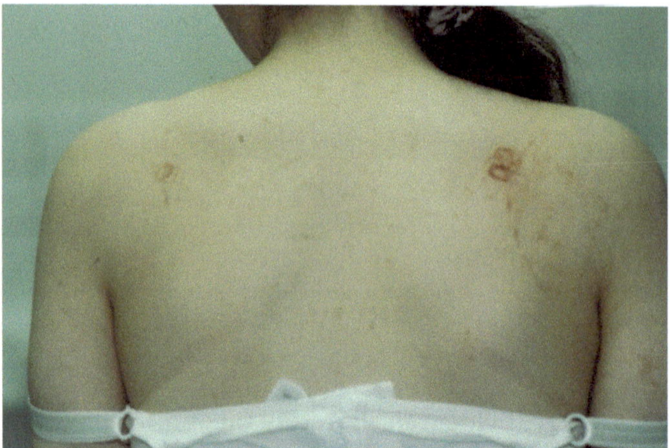

Fig. 9.3 Abutment injury: formed intracutaneous bleeding caused by pressure on the bra

outpatient department, they are mentioned here for the sake of completeness.

For adequate evidence recovery and further laboratory diagnostics, a larger number of samples must be taken:

In case of penetration, vaginal/rectal/oral swabs to detect semen and perpetrator DNA. Swabs should also be taken when a condom is used, as the ingredient Lycopodium can be detected.

In the case of bite injuries, also swabs for DNA detection from dried saliva.

Removal and cataloguing of adhering traces such as soil, hair, skin scales. For this purpose, the victim is placed in lithotomy position and then the pubic hair is combed out. The comb is also taken to the laboratory. The fingernails should be cut and examined because of possible adhering skin scales of the perpetrator after defensive measures.

All swabs and other specimens are individually sterile and dry packaged and accurately labeled.

From a laboratory chemistry point of view, a determination of the blood alcohol or drug level as well as a drug screening should be carried out, for which a blood sample and a urine sample are necessary. The blood sample can also be used to obtain the victim's DNA, which can then be used to identify any foreign DNA. Furthermore, a pregnancy test and serological tests for sexually transmitted diseases (STD) should be carried out at the same time.

Of course, the clothing is also examined by the investigating authorities for semen or saliva adhesions as well as clothing fibers or hair of the suspect.

9.3.5.4 Perpetrator Investigation

Not only the investigation of the victim, but also that of the alleged perpetrator can be ordered according to § 81a StPO. The suspect cannot evade this obligation and he cannot refuse any part of the investigation. The focus of interest is on evidence of defensive injuries of the victim, obtaining a DNA sample of the suspect as well as swabs (especially the shaft of the penis) or scraping off possible skin particles under the fingernails with the intention of proving the DNA of the victim.

9.3.5.5 Simulated Sexual Offence

It is known that 5–12% of all sexual offences reported to the police are faked.

This is particularly common in the age group of young girls up to 16 years, at around 40%.

The motivation for a false report can be exemplary:

- Justification for long absences, etc.
- Obtaining attention/care
- Revenge against the alleged perpetrator (~1/4 of the cases)
- hiding an infidelity

Not infrequently, this pretense is also associated with self-inflicted injuries. These injuries often have a characteristic shape and can thus serve to clarify the alleged offence: They are mostly grouped, parallel, uniform, often long-stretched, superficial injuries of the skin in symmetrical expression. They are localized on easily accessible parts of the body, painful regions are left out.

Certain sexual practices can be more easily used to fake a sexual offence, even though they were originally consensual.

Not to be confused with a forcible bondage to fixate the victim is the sexual bondage. In this case there is usually a strict parallelism and cleanliness of the loop, which is only possible because "the victim" does not resist. Another indication is the bondage of irrelevant body parts.

Both voluntarily and forced can result in the toleration of sexually motivated violence, which can be difficult to distinguish in court. Bites to the neck, mammary glands, abdomen, buttocks or thighs are sexually motivated. Likewise, there may be the insertion of objects into body orifices or "experimental" injuries.

It is very important to detect any false charges, as a conviction would have unjustified severe consequences for the alleged perpetrator and he has little chance to prove his innocence.

When approached and questioned about the suspicion of filing a false report, the persons concerned usually admit to their crime.

9.4 Child Abuse

9.4.1 Casuistry

You are alerted as an ambulance team in the evening hours to a terraced housing estate with the emergency message "Scalded child". The apartment door is opened by a man who claims to be the father of the two-year-old child. On his way into the bathroom he says that he feels very guilty because he accidentally put the child in the bathtub which was too hot. The little boy is awake and responsive, but seems very calm and withdrawn despite the great pain that is assumed. He looks sceptically at the arriving rescue team. Approximately 30% one- to two-degree scalds appear on both legs and on the trunk up to about the navel. While intravenous pain therapy is initiated and the wounds are sterilely covered, you ask the father about pre-existing conditions and the name of the attending pediatrician. You are told of several hospitals where the child had been treated for accidental injuries, that there was no permanent paediatrician in private practice, that they would always consult the nearest paediatrician if necessary. You inform the father that the child has to be treated as an in-patient in the children's hospital, which is initially met with displeasure, then with neutral agreement. When asked, you learn that the mother would take care of the two other siblings, aged 4 years and 3 months, who are already asleep.

You are not sure whether it is actually an accident or a deliberate scalding of the little boy. Do you leave the clarification of the facts to the admitting paediatrician, should you inform the police or should you approach the father or even the child about the suspicion? Uncertain, you decide on pure emergency medical treatment on the spot and rapid transport to the children's hospital. Once there, you speak to the admitting pediatrician about your suspicions. Somewhat irritated, he tells you that you have to take care of it if you have a suspicion, he would not accuse the parents without having seen the domestic situation. He could only say that the child had already been treated three times as an outpatient for bruises and a lower leg fracture. When asked again, the pediatrician agrees to initiate further clarification. You make detailed notes about your observations and impressions at the scene, as you are prepared for questioning by the police. Unsatisfied with the many unanswered questions, you leave the paediatric clinic.

9.4.2 Introduction

The subject of child abuse is a very sensitive area. As a professional helper, you want to bring all cases that come to your attention to clarification and possibly also to punishment. Every adult has a special sense of responsibility for children and children are generally considered vulnerable and defenseless. Reports of child abuse leave people speechless and often make them aware of their own powerlessness. On the other hand, there is a great risk of harm, which should not be underestimated, from an unjustified suspicion or one made in the wrong place. One must be aware of the far-reaching consequences that an investigation in such an area entails: the suspects will probably never seek professional help again in the event of a possible repetition, there is the threat of severe criminal consequcnces, families can break up and the job can be lost in the event of a suspicion. If a corresponding investigation becomes public, the social fabric in the place of residence, in the circle of friends and the family is often irreparably disturbed – not infrequently there is then talk of character assassination. The legal consequences, in addition to the crime suffered, also have consequences for the child concerned. Since the perpetrator in most cases comes from the close personal environment of the child, the child is taken out of this social structure and thus loses its attachment figures despite the damage suffered.

The decision as to where child abuse begins is not the responsibility of the emergency services, but may confidently be left to the courts. On the contrary, emergency medicine is responsible for a no less important descriptive task.

Prudent action and profound prior knowledge on the part of the rescue team can help to ensure that cases of abuse are uncovered; on the other hand, it saves innocent suspects from unwarranted consequences.

9.4.2.1 Definition and Forms of Child Abuse

Maltreatment is an act that causes possible or actual harm or exposes the child to the risk of harm. The act is volitional; the harm need not be intentional. Neglect is an act of omission. (Def. of the Centers for Disease Control and Prevention/CDC).

A distinction is made between the following types of child abuse, which affect those working in emergency medicine to varying degrees. Since the English terminology is often used, this is listed separately for the individual forms:

- Emotional abuse
- Neglect
- Physical abuse (child abuse)
- Sexual child abuse
- Medical child abuse (Munchausen-by-proxy-syndrome)

In the majority of cases, children are victims of more than one type of abuse; nevertheless, all forms are presented separately below for the sake of better differentiation and their specific characteristics.

9.4.3 Emotional Abuse

Emotional abuse of children is not uncommon, also in German-speaking countries. Nevertheless, there are hardly any corresponding statistics, as there is no uniform definition or criteria for this type of abuse. Where does a not particularly loving or authoritarian-strict upbringing end and where does emotional abuse begin? This leads to a lack of awareness of the problem in society. Often the cases of abuse are not recognized at all or not infrequently come to light only in adolescence or adulthood, for example in the context of psychotherapeutic treatments.

The following are some examples of possible forms of emotional abuse and appropriate references:

- Lack of loving attention: Children seem withdrawn and quiet. In the presence of the parents, the child does not show an attitude of trust towards the parents or it courts affection from the parents (perhaps this is what led to the rescue mission in the first place).

- Indications of deprivation of liberty: no child-friendly accommodation (e.g. confinement in a hutch).
- Threats: Child shows fear and reports inadequate consequences for misbehavior when asked.

Since such emotional maltreatment does not usually lead to a rescue service call, it is not particularly relevant to emergency physicians, especially since one cannot gather many clues or adequately assess them given the short contact time with the child.

9.4.4 Neglect

In principle, neglect does not have to be accompanied by emotional abuse, but there is a relatively high rate of coincidence. In the context of neglect, the child is not given the appropriate physical care and nurturing. For example, this may involve the hygienic conditions of the placement, extended personal hygiene, or nutrition. In addition, lack of supervision can lead to otherwise preventable problems. Nevertheless, this form is also difficult to grasp, since even children growing up in optimal conditions can be presented to the emergency services as patients, filthy and in torn clothes, after an adventure game in the woods resulting in accidental injury.

Nevertheless, suspicious facts should be pointed out, which should lead to a closer inspection, especially if they are present at the same time:

- Significantly too low age-appropriate weight
- Infectious skin diseases due to lack of personal hygiene (not chickenpox!)
- Extremely poor dental status
- Matted as well as otherwise unkempt hair
- Extremely long or torn fingernails and toenails
- Any evidence of disease due to malnutrition
- Poor spatial-material conditions (think, for example, of media reports about "children's rooms" in hovels, stables, etc.), which cannot be due to low income of the parents.

Often, cases of neglect come to light because when the age-appropriate percentile curves are drawn up, it becomes apparent that the child is not developing as expected in terms of height and weight. However, it is not possible to assess this in an emergency setting because both the instruments and the necessary time are lacking. Nevertheless, the small patients should be compared with children of the same age from the own family or the circle of acquaintances. In case of gross discrepancies, an inpatient evaluation is recommended not only because of the suspicion of neglect but also because of the suspicion of failure to thrive.

Even if physical or emotional violence is not actively used in neglect, physical or psychological damage (sometimes lifelong) can still occur.

9.4.5 Physical Abuse

9.4.5.1 Statistics

According to the Police Crime Statistics for Germany, 4100 children were affected by violent crimes in 2019, of which 2333 were boys and 1767 were girls. 1737 of the abused children were under 6 years old, while the remaining 2363 were between 6 and 14 years old. The clearance rate is very high at 97.4%, which is due to the fact that charges are usually not filed until a suspect is known. It is worth noting that 45.6% of the suspects are female.

In clear contrast to these rather low figures are the evaluations of the so-called 8a reports. These are all cases of suspected child welfare endangerment that are reported to the youth welfare office. Here, 157,300 reports were reviewed by the youth welfare office in 2019. Of these, 24,900 reports were seen to pose an acute risk to the welfare of the child, and a further 25,500 were seen to pose a latent risk to the welfare of the child. What about the remaining 2/3 of the reports? In a further third (around 53,000) no risk to the welfare of the child was identified, but a general need for help on the part of the families to prevent a later escalation; this includes, for example, educational counselling or socio-educational family support. In the last third of the reports, neither a risk to the welfare of the child nor a need for help was seen by the youth welfare office. This large number of "false interventions" is due, among other things, to the fact that when custodians separate, the accusation of maltreatment or abuse is quickly made without there being any real maltreatment.

9.4.5.2 Criminology

Young children (2.–4 years of age) are particularly at risk of becoming victims of physical abuse. Approximately 75% of cases involve children before the age of 7. If several children grow up together in one family, it is not uncommon that only one child is affected. The perpetrators usually come from the children's immediate environment, such as parents or stepparents. In most cases, there is a chronic recurrent course, in which, however, escalations can occur.

9.4.5.3 Forms of Physical Abuse

The following forms can be roughly distinguished, which will be discussed in more detail below:

(a) Blunt force
   - Blows with hand, fist or tools
   - Bumping into furniture or walls
   - Kicks
(b) Bite
(c) Bonds

(d) Burning/scalding
(e) Hypothermia
(f) Near suffocation
(g) Poison
(h) Shaking of newborns/infants and young children

Blunt Force

Blunt force is usually used with the hand or fist, but a tool (e.g. belt, rope, stick) can also be used (Fig. 9.5). Children can also be pushed against fixed objects such as furniture or walls or down the stairs. Last but not least, kicking injuries should also be mentioned. In terms of differential diagnosis, accident-related injuries should be considered first and foremost. Some clues can help to distinguish between accident and abuse. First of all, the localization of the injuries: In Fig. 9.4, one can see which sites are typically involved when a child trips and falls (without an obstacle), and which sites require more detailed explanation. For example, a hematoma on the abdomen cannot be explained by a simple fall, but is plausible if it is reported that the child fell on a box in the process. Also suspicious are so-called shaped injuries where the causative objects are apparent, for example edges or loops. A third clue may be the number and grouping; abuse-related hematomas are typically seen in large numbers and grouped together (Fig. 9.5).

Bite

Bite wounds (Fig. 9.6), although usually not vitally threatening, can be very painful and are a special kind of humiliation for the victim. There is a great risk of infection in the case of open wounds. When inspecting an alleged bite wound, pay particular attention to any tooth marks and, in the case of open wounds, to substance defects. Tooth marks are also of interest when an animal bite wound is pretended. As a rough guide, bite wounds with tissue injuries are more likely to be of animal origin due to the sharp points of animal teeth (cats/dogs) and in human bite wounds hematomas can be seen in the form of two half arches. The diameter of these half arches can give an indication of whether a child, for example in play, or an adult has bitten. Child dentitions

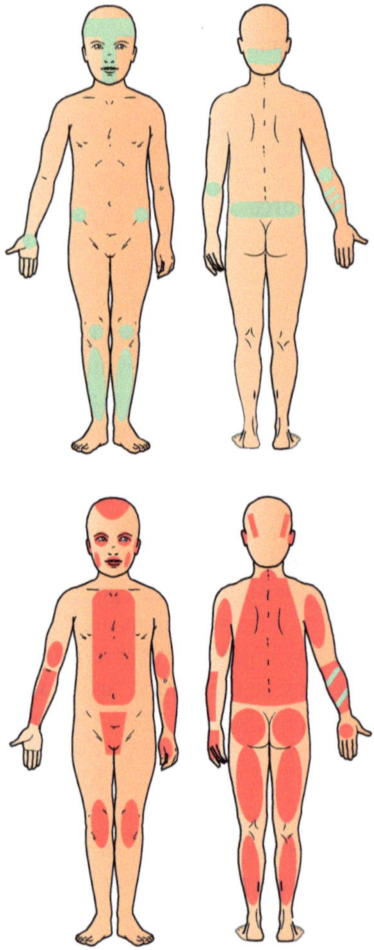

Fig. 9.4 Typical locations when a child drops and falls (green) and untypical locations (red)

before the change of teeth typically have a diameter < 2.5 cm, adults of more than 3 cm. In the case of bites in the context of sexual abuse, petechiae may also occur in the interior of the hematoma arches due to sucking by the perpetrator.

Bonds

Children are restrained either to "immobilize" them or to directly harm them physically. In addition to the actual restriction of

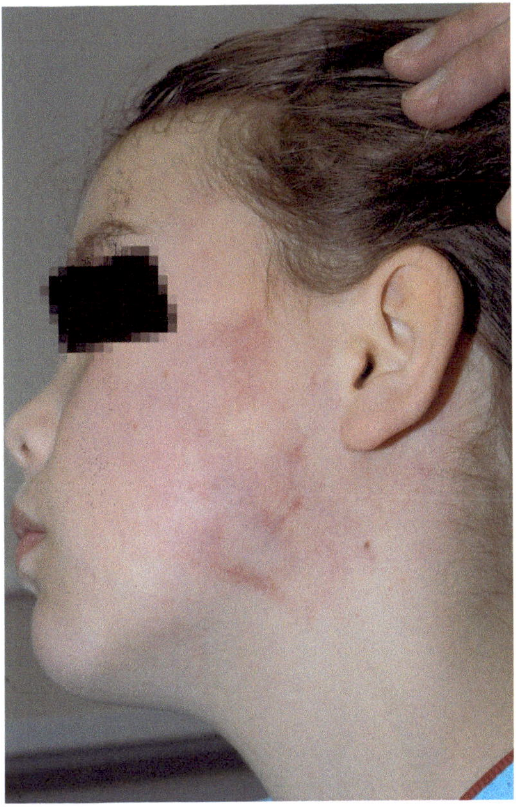

Fig. 9.5 Partially formed skin hemorrhages of the left side of the face after multiple blows, partly with objects

self-determined mobility, this can also lead to further damage such as restrictions on breathing. Physical signs that restraint has taken place may be absent or very discrete. The most likely signs are band-like hematomas or superficial abrasions. Very thin materials may result in deeper, cut-like wounds. Attention should be paid to the circular nature of the injuries.

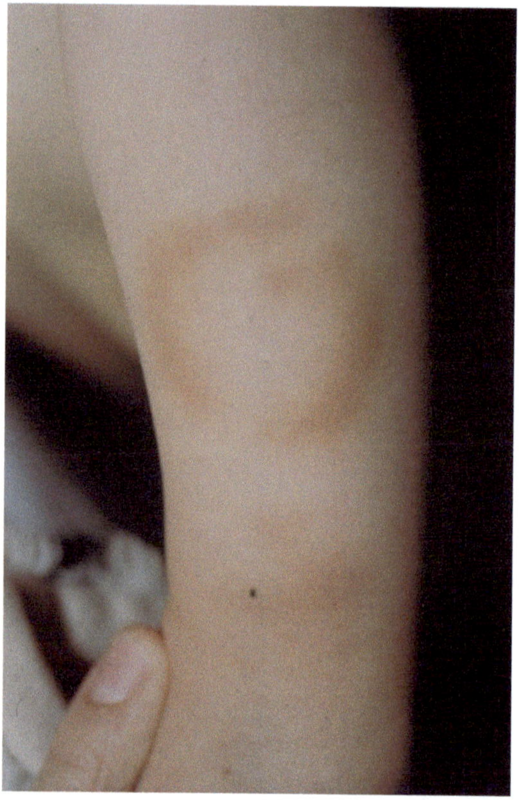

Fig. 9.6 Bite marks on the upper arm

Burning/Scalding

With regard to determining the extent and severity of heat injury, reference should be made to the separate chapter of this book (Sect. 5.5). In the context of child abuse, it is mostly small-surface, clearly localizable burns caused, for example, by cigarettes or by pressing on other hot objects (iron, cooking pot, hotplate, etc.) Abuse-related scalding is rarely an overpouring with hot liquid – this is also hardly distinguishable from accidental overpouring – but rather a forced immersion in liquids that are too hot. The feet

± lower legs, arms ± forearms or the whole child are forced into the hot liquid and fixed in this position. These scalds are easier to distinguish from accidents because there are clear boundaries between damaged and uninjured skin and hardly any secondary injuries. A child who accidentally reaches into a liquid that is too hot would immediately withdraw the arm, the boundary to scalding would be blurred, and there would be small scalds in the surrounding area from the splashes of water.

Undercool

Unlike burns/scalds, hypothermia is usually not a localized injury. Children are locked in cold ambient air or immersion in cold liquids takes place. The exposure time to detectable injury is significantly longer than heat exposure. Apart from the measurable reduction in body temperature a short time after exposure to cold, there is often no physical evidence, which significantly limits the burden of proof. It should be emphasized, however, that no physical signs are necessary for the facts of the case.

Near Suffocation

The intention behind this use of force can range from the aim of "immobilising" a crying child to humiliation through the display of power. In addition to holding the breathing orifices shut or choking, instruments such as cords, ropes, gags, but also pillows are used. Problematic with the use of soft objects are the discrete injuries, which can make the proof very difficult.

Poison

Again, the perpetrator may have the goal of sedating the child by administering sedating substances. Unfortunately, deliberate harm to health may also occur through the use of drugs, chemicals, or plant parts. In Munchausen by proxy syndrome, which will be discussed later in the chapter, children are sometimes poisoned in order to cause symptoms of illness, such as vague unconsciousness, vomiting, diarrhoea, etc. The perpetrator may also use drugs to sedate the child.

Abusive Head Injuries: Abusive Head Trauma

This umbrella term covers all injuries to the head caused by maltreatment. For the most part, these are children with shaking trauma syndrome, but also injuries caused by the child hitting the floor or a wall.

Shaking baby syndrome mainly affects infants at the prime crying age, i.e. from 2 to 5 months. During shaking, the child is grasped by the trunk or upper arms and moved violently back and forth several times in an upright position. Due to the not yet strongly developed neck and neck musculature, small children are not able to hold their head independently, which is disproportionately large in comparison to adults, and certainly not during whiplash movements of the trunk. This results in a translational trauma of the brain with the following possible consequences (in each case not a must!): subdural haemorrhage, diffuse axonal damage (encephalopathy), cerebral oedema and pronounced retinal haemorrhages. Children may appear very different depending on the severity and duration of the shaking. Some show few symptoms, such as general irritability, weakness in drinking, vomiting, while others are floppy, unconscious, show gasping for breath and may require resuscitation. In unconscious children up to kindergarten age, a possible shaking trauma should always be considered, at least as a differential diagnosis, in addition to intoxication. As a rule, there are no external signs of injuries that are serious or even fatal in themselves – only sometimes are there traces of grasping on the upper arms or torso. Radiological examinations of the head (acute cCT, after stabilization MRI to show cerebral edema and subdural hemorrhage) and of the chest (rib fractures, especially dorsally localized) are indicated to establish the diagnosis. Retinal hemorrhage can be seen on fundoscopy. About a quarter of affected children die and of those who survive, about 75% show permanent damage.

9.4.5.4 Suspicions

Of course, it is not possible to provide any binding information or instructions here as to which signs of physical violence should be investigated further or the police should be called in. Nevertheless, it is possible to identify circumstances which, even in the case of a short period of contact such as an ambulance call, represent indications of physical abuse, even if this is far from being proven:

- Missing, vague, unclear or changing explanations about the course of the accident
- (Serious) injuries allegedly inflicted by siblings (injuries inflicted by siblings are common, but most are not serious compared to violence inflicted by adults)
- Accident mechanism inadequate for age/developmental state
- Delay in seeking medical help (the child was injured the day before, but the ambulance service is only now being called).
- Discovery of additional unreported injuries (possibly of different ages) on physical examination.
- Repeated injuries with frequent change of doctor
- Information from third parties or from the child itself
- Localisation: Suspicious for maltreatment are injuries on cheeks, ears, back, buttocks, back of legs (Figs. 9.4 and 9.7). Unsuspicious are injuries above the knee joints, on the elbows and on the front of the lower legs. Highly suspicious of abuse are sock- or glove-like scalds

In addition, one should always ask oneself the following question: Could the child have self-inflicted the injuries due to motor skills?

9.5 Sexual Abuse of Children

9.5.1 Statistics

The 2019 police crime statistics Germany record **13,670** cases of child sexual abuse. Note that this is significantly more cases than for physical abuse. However, this says nothing about the frequency distribution of the respective crimes, but it is a reflection of the fact that sexual assault may be reported more quickly than physical abuse. Eighty-seven per cent of child sexual offences

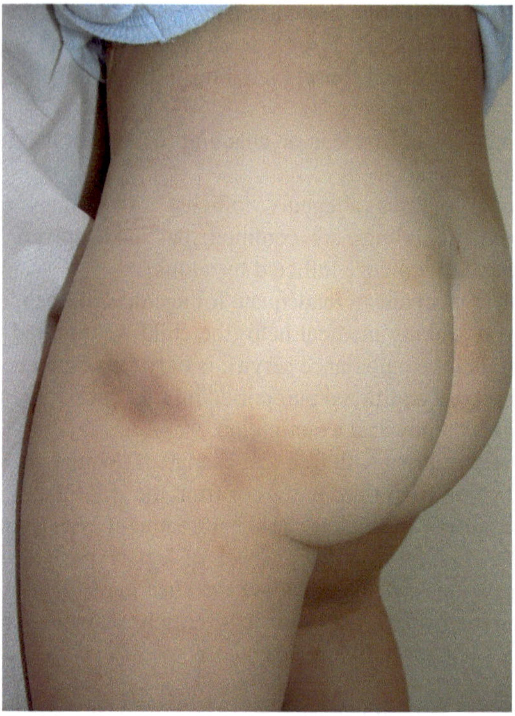

Fig. 9.7 Haematomas resulting from blows to the buttocks

reported to the police were solved in 2019. Of the 10,259 suspects, 93% were male, showing that in the majority of cases, men are the perpetrators in sexual abuse, but women can become perpetrators too! Girls accounted for 75% of the 15,701 victims. There was a significant increase in cases of distribution, acquisition, possession and production of child pornography to 12,262 cases in 2019.

The above-mentioned statistical surveys of the investigating authorities should not hide the fact that the number of unreported cases is much higher. In a large-scale study in Germany in 2016, 13.9% of respondents (all age groups) stated that they had been victims of child sexual abuse in the past. Similarly, the statistics of the Federal Criminal Police Office do not reflect the fact that in a high percentage of cases it does not remain with a one-time sexual assault, but it is often a course of years with the possibility of escalation.

As an emergency medical technician, it is important to remember that the ambulance service is called to only a fraction of child sex offences.

9.5.2 Visible Consequences/Problems of Detection

Only in very rare cases is a sexual offence in children provable by means of a physical examination, as normal physical findings can be obtained in about 90% of cases. Similarly, there is no specific abuse syndrome. Any physical findings are to be evaluated only in connection with the child's statement.

In many cases there are no visible indications of sexual abuse, and examples of this can be found here:

- Sexual acts without penetration
  - genital touching
  - Viewing the genitals
  - Insertion of thin objects such as fingers
- Allowing the child to perform sexual acts
- pornography show

But even if penetration has occurred, the high regeneration potential of the anogenital tissue means that any injuries cannot be seen or can only be seen shortly after the act.

The following physical consequences of sexual assault may be apparent:

Injuries in the genital, anal and/or oral area, as well as possibly in other parts of the body, bite-suck injuries, foreign bodies in the urethra, bladder, vagina or anus. The injuries may be *very discrete or even absent.* Injuries heal very quickly in children, so early documentation and attestation is important.

9.5.3 Diagnostics

Apart from a vital danger to the victim, an examination and questioning of the child should only be carried out in an adequate environment, by experienced personnel (of both sexes) and after sufficient material preparation, and is therefore clearly not the responsibility of the emergency services. Maximum reverence and empathy should be ensured. If possible, the child should be made to endure a full body inspection including the anogenital area. An examination that is not carried out by an examiner experienced in this (if possible a paediatric gynaecologist) carries the risk of re-traumatising the child due to the similar position to that of the abuse that took place. For the rescue service, on the other hand, it is important to preserve any clothing, nappies, etc. for further tracing. Swabs for trace analysis should be taken as early as possible, at least within 72 h.

The questioning also requires an experienced examiner: A careful anamnesis with age-adapted open questions has to take place. The history should be documented exactly, if possible verbatim (who asked how, how did the child answer). Suggestive questioning is to be avoided at all costs. Spontaneous accusations are to be taken seriously in the first place, because concrete false accusations are rare. Repeated questioning is to be avoided. Since there is neither the time for extensive questioning nor the experience in this particular subject in the emergency service, questioning of the child should be avoided. If the child talks of his or her own accord because he/she feels the need to confide in someone, let him/her talk, signal sympathy but preferably no fright, indignation or grief, etc., and refrain from asking follow-up questions. All statements should be documented as verbatim as possible.

9.6 Medical Child Abuse/Factitious Disorder Imposed on Another (FDIA)

Factitious disorder imposed on another (FDIA) formerly called Munchausen by proxy syndrom is a special case of child abuse. In this case, an illness of the child is feigned by third parties (mostly the parents and predominantly by the mothers) through physical manipulation of any kind. For example, medication such as diuretics or laxatives may be administered, or pre-existing wounds may be manipulated in such a way that they heal poorly. The intention for the act is usually a hoped-for secondary gain in illness for the perpetrator through increased affection and attention from third parties – either in the closer personal environment or as a way of calling for help from public authorities in the event of being overwhelmed with childcare. Medical child abuse is rarely known or proven beyond doubt, yet it must be suspected that this abuse entity is not a rarity.

9.7 Medical Child Protection Hotline

The medical child protection hotline has been in place since summer 2017 (see Fig. 9.8). Here, doctors from the fields of paediatrics, child and adolescent psychiatry and forensic medicine work as telephone advisors for all medical professions on questions relating to child protection. This can be, for example, the

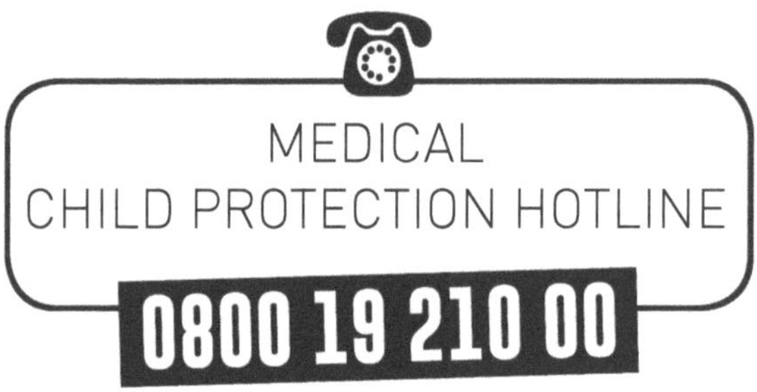

Fig. 9.8 Medical child protection hotline

physiotherapist who has noticed haematomas and now does not know whether and how to proceed. Or the ambulance worker who is unsure whether the observations they have made in the field are suspicious and how to proceed. Since child protection cannot be planned, the hotline is staffed 24 h/day, 365 days/year. The hotline is free of charge for the caller, as it is currently funded by the Federal Ministry of Family Affairs. The patient data remains anonymous, if the caller wants it, the caller can also remain anonymous. The hotline is supposed to be a low-threshold offer to consult among colleagues before approaching the youth welfare office or the police, especially if one is still unsure.

9.8 Further Information and Assistance Possibilities

If you would like to learn more about the subject of child abuse, you can find numerous publications on the Internet from various professional societies, or you can read the relevant specialist books.

On statistical questions for Germany, the Federal Criminal Police Office can help with the police crime statistics on the one hand, but also the Federal Statistical Office, which gives the figures of the assessments of the risk to the welfare of children by the Youth Welfare Office.

There is also help for the victims and their relatives, here are just a few examples: Weißer Ring, Nummer gegen Kummer, Hilfetelefon sexueller Missbrauch, Wildwasser, Telefonseelsorge. All the mentioned examples are for Germany.

For people who are considering reporting to the Youth Welfare Service, there is also the “ISeF”, the experienced specialist, who can help from the side of the Youth Welfare Service to decide whether there is a risk to the well-being of the child or not. The counselling here is pseudonymous.

Toxicology 10

10.1 Case Histories

On a sultry summer evening, you as the Paramedic team are called to a reported unconscious person in a middle-class home. There you are welcomed by the panic-stricken wife with the words "I think it's too late" and led into the basement workshop. There, in the middle of the workshop, lies an approx. 50-year-old man in a lateral position. No signs of life can be detected, the pupils are distended and, on closer inspection, incipient postmortem lividity can be made out. Therefore, you refrain from resuscitation efforts. There is a conspicuous dried trace of vomit from one corner of the mouth and a small puddle of what is presumably vomit next to the deceased. There is an open empty fizzy drink bottle without a label on the workbench from which a pungent odor is emanating. The wife states that her husband had retired to carpentry on the old dresser – he had been somewhat introverted lately, which she attributed to the loss of his job 3 months ago.

You tell the woman emotionally that you have to inform the police because of the unexplained manner of death, as you suspect that the man drank from the bottle and it is not clear to you what the content was and whether it was accidental (perhaps hasty due to the sultry weather) or suicidal ingestion.

As you fill out the death certificate, you consider how the police or coroner can resolve the outstanding issues.

S. Ahne et al., *Forensic aspects in emergency medicine*,
https://doi.org/10.1007/978-3-662-65949-6_10

10.2 Introduction

Poisoning is one of the most common causes of death. The cause of death statistics Germany show 1120 deaths from accidental intoxications in 2018. Drugs and medicines dominate among the substances, fatal poisonings by gases such as carbon monoxide or carbon dioxide, corrosives or metals are rarer.

The very extensive subject of poisoning can only be touched upon briefly and by way of example here. Non-fatal courses are much more frequent than fatal ones and are therefore dealt with much more frequently in emergency medicine. The diagnosis of fatal poisoning can only be made by toxicological examinations following an autopsy. However, the circumstances in which a corpse is found, the external findings during post-mortem examination and the internal findings can be diagnostic.

10.3 External Findings of the Corpse

During the external postmortem examination, numerous findings may be indicative of intoxication. Light red livor mortis occur in cases of poisoning by carbon monoxide or cyanides, and brownish grey livor mortis in cases of poisoning by nitrates. Vomit is often found around the respiratory openings (Fig. 10.1). In addition to vomit, a bloody foam fungus is sometimes noticeable. This may occur in poisoning as a result of haemorrhagic pulmonary oedema, particularly in cases of drug death, but also in other intoxications if they are accompanied by prolonged hypoxia. Since this foam fungus can easily be destroyed during transport of the corpse and does not always re-emerge, it should definitely be documented.

The smell can give clues to the ingested agent. In the case of prolonged agonal recumbency, pressure marks, and/or characteristic skin blisters (so-called HOLZER's blisters) may appear where the body rested on the ground (Fig. 10.2). As such, the main areas to be mentioned are: Thigh/hip region, inner sides of knees, ankles, dorsum of fingers, dorsum of toes or spine.

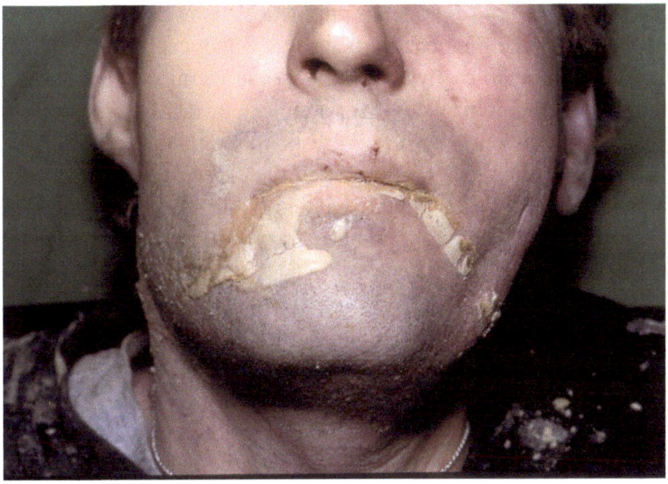

Fig. 10.1 Vomiting at the mouth in case of fatal drug intoxication

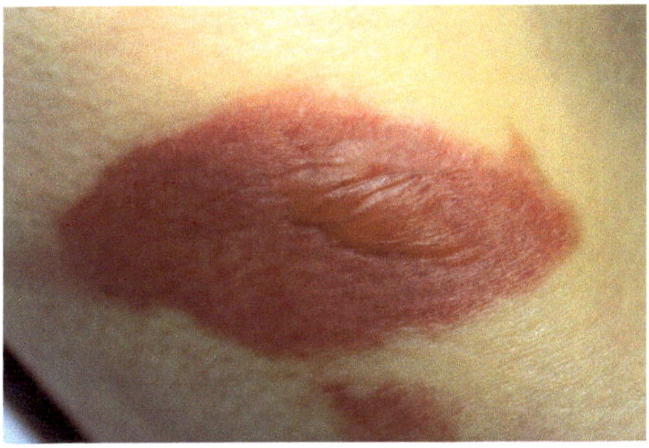

Fig. 10.2 Holzer's blister: pressure-induced skin blister after prolonged agony in the context of fatal intoxication

Likewise, prolonged premortem recumbency often results in urinary leakage. Such recumbencies, sometimes lasting several hours, are by no means uncommon in fatal intoxications. Also, occasionally the body is found in a somewhat hidden position, such as under the table or under the bed, which at first glance may be suspicious of extraneous influence. However, it can be explained by the final caving behavior, which can also occur, for example, in death by hypothermia. In the vicinity of the corpse, (empty) medicine packets, fixer's cutlery or drinking containers with adhesions may provide corresponding clues (Fig. 10.3). In order to facilitate the clarification of the cause of death, the findings should also be documented and possibly preserved and given to the corpse, such as the alleged fizzy drink bottle in the case example.

10.4 Internal Findings of the Corpse

There are few specific internal cadaver findings in intoxications. Typical but non-specific for intoxications is the combination of cerebral edema, pulmonary edema, blood stasis of the internal organs, aspiration of stomach contents and full urinary bladder. Depending on the substance, other internal changes may occur:

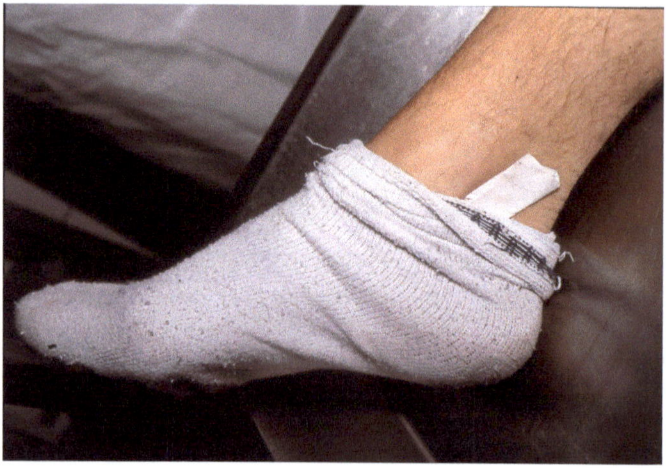

Fig. 10.3 Heroin packet hidden on the body in a sock

Drugs: Injection needle marks through veins, hemorrhagic pulmonary edema ...

Carbon monoxide: Salmon red discoloration of the muscles, light red cadaveric blood ...

Medication: Partially dissolved tablets in the contents of the stomach

Corrosive: burns in the upper gastrointestinal tract, in case of aspiration also in the bronchi

10.5 Drugs and Medication

In cases of drug-related deaths, in addition to the above-mentioned signs of a prolonged phase of agony, further findings may frequently be encountered. A typical finding is a forward bent to crouching posture. In the presence of hemorrhagic pulmonary edema, copious amounts of bloody fluid may passively drain from

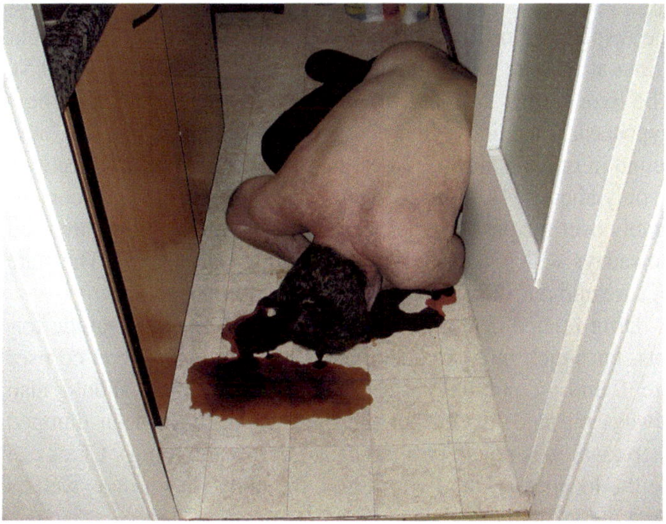

Fig. 10.4 Fatal heroin intoxication. Typical is the bent-over, crouching posture

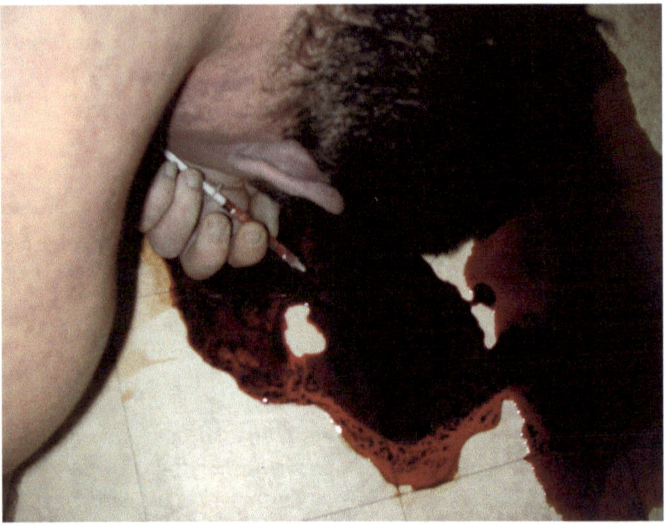

Fig. 10.5 Discharge of bloody fluid from the respiratory orifices as a result of the head down position in haemorrhagic pulmonary oedema

the respiratory orifices, which may raise suspicion of a violent crime at the site where the body is found (Figs. 10.4 and 10.5). The livor mortis are very often intensely pronounced and show hypostasis bleeding (vibices). Fresh injection marks are now found in only about 60% of cases, scars from repeated injections in only about 50%. The spectrum of findings has changed considerably over the past decades. As a rule, insulin injections are used nowadays which cause hardly any visible skin lesions. The state of care and nutrition is now also mostly normal.

Drug-related deaths are nowadays rarely found in public toilets, but much more frequently in private homes. When corpses are found in publicly accessible areas, attention should also always be paid to whether the corpse may have been dumped there, which is not so rare (so-called corpse dumping). Clues can be the location of the livor mortis, the body's posture as well as drag marks on the body and in the surrounding area.

Monointoxications, e.g. by heroin, are rather rare nowadays. Mostly, they are mixed intoxications by opiates, other drugs, alcohol, benzodiazepines, amphetamines and medicines.

Pure drug poisoning usually occurs with suicidal intent. Psychotropic drugs are the most commonly used, but cardiac drugs or insulin are also repeatedly used for suicidal purposes.

10.6 Carbon Monoxide

Carbon monoxide (CO) is a colourless and odourless gas which is lighter than air and is produced during the combustion of organic material. It has an affinity for the red blood pigment haemoglobin (Hb) that is about 250 times higher than oxygen. Even a room air concentration of more than 0.1% by volume can be fatal. Smokers may have a CO-Hb concentration of 6% in their blood. Values of more than 10% are considered signs of intoxication, with values above 50% being fatal in healthy adults. From about 20%, the first symptoms of poisoning are to be expected (headache, fatigue, dizziness), from about 30% lethargy and impaired consciousness are added.

The most important indication of fatal carbon monoxide poisoning at postmortem examination are the light red livor mortis. In contrast to the postmortem light red discoloration in the context of cold exposure, the livor mortis in CO intoxication are also light red under the fingernails and toenails, on the palms and soles of the feet. Zoning of the livor mortis with light red and livid portions as in cold exposure does not occur. Furthermore, the oral mucous membranes appear "fresh from life".

The possibility of CO intoxication should be considered even if a CO source is not obvious. For example, a garden barbecue that was brought into the house with the charcoals still glowing may have been moved aside by the original body finder.

10.7 Carbon Dioxide

The toxicity of the odourless and tasteless gas carbon dioxide (CO_2) is relatively low, but as it is heavier than air, it can accumulate in ground depressions, shafts, wells, fermentation cellars or silos. At concentrations greater than 8%, hyperventilation, headaches and dizziness occur. At more than 10%, respiratory paralysis, convulsions and then death occur.

The findings at necropsy are nonspecific. The hypostasis may be intense, possibly a reddish foam fungus is found in front of the respiratory openings as a sign of hemorrhagic pulmonary edema.

10.8 Cyanides

Cyanides and hydrocyanic acid are used in the precious metals industry and for surface hardening in metal processing. Furthermore, cyanides are released during fires of plastics. The substances are extremely toxic and are rapidly absorbed. When ingested orally, 1–2 mg HCN/kg body mass are lethal. Cyanides block cell respiration by binding to cytochrome oxidase.

A typical feature is the bitter almond odour, which can be detected both on the poison itself and on intoxicated persons, provided that the examiner is sensitive to this odour (genetically predisposed). The corpse examination may reveal light red livor mortis, which, however, are usually not as pronounced as in CO intoxication.

10.9 Caustic

Caustics are divided into acids and alkalis. Typical acids are hydrochloric acid (HCl), sulfuric acid (H_2SO_4), nitric acid (HNO_3) or organic acids such as acetic acid. Typical alkalis are sodium hydroxide (NaOH) or potassium hydroxide (KOH). Both acids and alkalis destroy tissue, with acids causing coagulation necrosis and alkalis causing colliquative necrosis. The latter are more dangerous because they are not self-limiting. Caustics may be taken both accidentally and suicidally. Furthermore, external administration occurs, for example, in the context of child abuse.

During the post-mortem examination, one usually already notices traces of cauterization on the mouth. If vomiting has occurred, then there are also corresponding burns on the respiratory orifices and dryness of the face in the places where the skin had contact with the agent.

10.10 Asservation

In cases of both survived and fatal intoxications or their suspected cases, it should be remembered to preserve drinking containers with contents or adhesions for toxicological investigations. A sample of vomit can also be preserved. Screwable plastic containers are suitable for this purpose. A blood sample (serum) and a urine sample can also be collected. However, this is not absolutely necessary in the case of deaths that come to a forensic post-mortem examination, as body fluids are retained for toxicological examinations in the course of the post-mortem examination anyway and no further decomposition takes place in the meantime.

Appendix

Recommended Reading

Ahne T, Mayer Scarnato W (2019) Komplikationen in der Notfallmedizin. Springer, Berlin

Birngruber C, Lasczkowski G, Dettmeyer R (2020) Forensische Verletzungskunde. Springer, Berlin

Dettmeyer R, Veit F, Verhoff M (2019) Rechtsmedizin, 3. Aufl. Springer, Berlin

Dirks B (2013) Die Notfallmedizin. Springer, Berlin

Fegert JM, Hoffmann U, König E, Niehues J, Liebhardt H (2015) Sexueller Missbrauch von Kindern und Jugendlichen. Springer, Berlin

Goldbeck L, Allrogen M, Münzer A, Rassenhofer M, Fegert JM (2017) Sexueller Missbrauch. Hogrefe, Göttingen

Grassberger M, Schmid H (2014) Todesermittlung. 2. Aufl. Wissenschaftliche Verlagsgesellschaft, Stuttgart

Grassberger M, Yen K, Türk E (2013) Klinisch-forensische Medizin. Springer, Berlin

Hammer U, Büttner A (2014) Leichenschau. Schattauer, Stuttgart

Herrmann B, Dettmeyer R, Banaschak S, Thyen U (2016) Kindesmisshandlung. 3. Aufl. Springer, Berlin

Keil W (2017) BASICS Rechtsmedizin, 3. Aufl. Elsevier, München

S. Ahne et al., *Forensic aspects in emergency medicine*,
https://doi.org/10.1007/978-3-662-65949-6

Madea B, Mußhoff F, Tag B (2012) Kurzlehrbuch Rechtsmedizin. Huber, Bern
Madea B (2019) Die ärztliche Leichenschau. Springer, Berlin
Musolff C, Hoffmann J (2006) Täterprofile bei Gewaltverbrechen, Springer, Berlin
Saukko P, Knight B (2016) Knight's forensic pathology, fourth edition, CRC Press, Boca Raton
Schön C, Wolf K (2019) Medizinische Akutversorgung nach sexualisierter Gewalt. Springer, Berlin

Internet

Institut für Rechtsmedizin der Universität Würzburg: https://www.med.uni-wuerzburg.de/rechtsmedizin/startseite/
Institut für Rechtsmedizin des Universitätsklinikums Freiburg: https://www.uniklinik-freiburg.de/rechtsmedizin.html
Untersuchungsstelle für Opfer häuslicher Gewalt, Rechtsmedizin München (Infomaterial, Dokumentationsbögen): https://www.rechtsmedizin.med.uni-muenchen.de/wissenschaft/klinische_rechtsmed/ambul_gewaltopfer/index.html
Deutsche Gesellschaft für Kinderschutz in der Medizin: https://www.dgkim.de/
Medizinische Kinderschutzhotline: https://www.kinderschutzhotline.de/
Passion Notfallmedizin: www.passion-notfallmedizin.de
News Papers – neue interessante wissenschaftliche Publikationen aus der Notfallmedizin: www.news-papers.eu
PINCAST – Perspektive Interdisziplinäre Notfallmedizin Podcast: www.pincast.net